"Regular rhythms are a mood stabilizer. If it makes sense to ta[...] to *do* social rhythm therapy (SRT). Not just learn about it, *do* [...] that's what you're holding, from one of the world's bipolar experts. As Holly Swartz says: [...] kind to yourself if you falter.' Become your own expert."

> —**Jim Phelps, MD**, founder of www.psycheducation.org, and author of *A Spectrum Approach to Mood Disorders* and *Why Am I Still Depressed?*

"If you or someone you care about has symptoms of bipolar disorder, this book is for you. It is a tour de force distillation of over two decades of clinical and research work that will help people understand their body clocks and how they can be empowered to improve their moods by strengthening their daily routines. Offering very user-friendly tools, this SRT workbook provides novel clinically and scientifically informed ways to feel better."

> —**Hilary Blumberg, MD**, Furth Professor of Psychiatric Neuroscience; professor of psychiatry, radiology, and child study; and director of the Mood Disorders Research Program at Yale School of Medicine

"Swartz has written an eminently readable book on the SRT approach, one of the few psychosocial interventions shown to be effective alongside of medications for bipolar disorder. Readers will learn how to keep their daily and nightly routines regulated, manage stressors that could disrupt routines, and minimize the frequency and severity of recurrences. Important reading for people seeking to enhance their quality of life with bipolar disorder."

> —**David J. Miklowitz, PhD**, distinguished professor of psychiatry and biobehavioral sciences in the Semel Institute for Neuroscience and Human Behavior at the University of California, Los Angeles; and author of *The Bipolar Disorder Survival Guide*

"Following decades of accomplished clinical practice and research, Holly Swartz expertly guides us in applying SRT principles to our lives. Swartz explains why and how modifying the timing of our daily routines and activities will improve our mood. Swartz enlightens us about circadian science—she is engaging and scientifically precise without being confusing! It's a standout how-to for anyone seeking better mental health and wellness through science."

> —**Danielle M. Novick, PhD**, director of the Outpatient Behavioral Health Interdisciplinary Program at Veterans Affairs Medical Center Pittsburgh, therapist, trainer, and member of the International Society of Interpersonal Psychotherapy

"Have you ever felt tired and not tired, or awake but not awake, at the same time? Swartz's book will help you to understand why. This book provides a straightforward explanation of daily rhythms and how they impact our body and mood, especially for individuals with bipolar disorder. You will find easy-to-use tools in this book to learn about your rhythms and how to improve them to feel better."

—**Louisa Sylvia, PhD**, associate director at the Dauten Family Center for Bipolar Treatment Innovation at Massachusetts General Hospital, author of *The Wellness Workbook for Bipolar Disorder*, and coauthor of *The Bipolar II Disorder Workbook*

"In her compassionate, wise, and powerful book, Holly Swartz has given those of us living with bipolar an unprecedented and life-changing gift. Swartz has a rare capacity to make cutting-edge brain science accessible to the rest of us, and then to translate those insights into actions we can take to maximize our health. I have lived with bipolar for over four decades: this is the only book I've found that gives us the tools we need to be at the helm, navigating our way to living in full vitality for the long term. Everyone living with bipolar should have a copy of *The Social Rhythm Therapy Workbook for Bipolar Disorder* on their shelf."

—**Sara Schley**, author of *BrainStorm*, and creator of the *BrainStorm* documentary

"As a bipolar survivor and thriver, setting disciplined social rhythms has been inextricable to my recovery journey. Professor Swartz, one of the world's foremost psychiatrists and researchers of bipolar disorder, gives tangible strategies to help identify, record, and track internal and external factors that significantly impact mental health. This brilliant workbook is a powerful tool and a must for anyone wanting to manage their moods and take better control of their life."

—**Maj. Gen. Gregg F. Martin, PhD, US Army (Retired)**, author of *Bipolar General*

"We know from research, clinical, and lived experience expertise that stabilizing body clocks and social rhythms is a powerful route to health and wellness in people living with bipolar disorder. Now, for the first time, we have an accessible, evidence-based, and comprehensive workbook designed to put this knowledge and concrete tools directly into the hands of people with the condition."

—**Erin Michalak, PhD**, professor of psychiatry at the University of British Columbia in Canada, expert in collaborative bipolar disorder research, and director of CREST.BD

The Social Rhythm Therapy Workbook for Bipolar Disorder

Stabilize Your Circadian Rhythms to Reduce Stress, Manage Moods, and Prevent Future Episodes

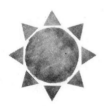   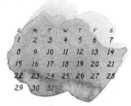

HOLLY A. SWARTZ, MD

New Harbinger Publications, Inc.

Publisher's Note

NEW HARBINGER PUBLICATIONS is a registered trademark of New Harbinger Publications, Inc.

New Harbinger Publications is an employee-owned company.

Copyright © 2024 by Holly A. Swartz
New Harbinger Publications, Inc.
5720 Shattuck Avenue
Oakland, CA 94609
www.newharbinger.com

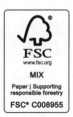

Printed in the United States of America

26   25   24

10   9   8   7   6   5   4   3   2   1   First Printing

This book is dedicated to my favorite social zeitgebers—
Steven, Sophie, Eli, Nellie Lou, Susie, and Peter.

Contents

Foreword

Dr. Holly Swartz's impressive volume, *The Social Rhythm Therapy Workbook for Bipolar Disorder: Stabilize Your Circadian Rhythms to Reduce Stress, Manage Moods, and Prevent Future Episodes*, fills a critical gap in the effort to bring the benefits of social rhythm therapy (SRT) to the broadest possible audience. Although medications are the foundation of bipolar disorder management, behavioral treatments are an essential part of care. This workbook will provide you with behavioral strategies you can use to better manage your moods. You will learn to identify, track, and create regular daily routines—a scientifically proven way of enhancing mood stability. Each chapter provides knowledgeable tips and exercises to facilitate your journey to wellness.

When I developed interpersonal and social rhythm therapy, the progenitor of SRT, almost thirty years ago, I could not have predicted how relevant it would become. The circadian basis of bipolar disorder has emerged as one of the most plausible explanations for the illness. A growing body of evidence underscores the importance of circadian rhythm regularity for those with mood disorders and, indeed, many other health conditions. Thus, a workbook on SRT is both timely and well aligned with existing knowledge about circadian rhythms and health.

Dr. Swartz and I routinely receive requests from therapists around the world who want to be trained in this treatment approach so that they can offer it to their patients. We also receive numerous requests from individuals living with bipolar disorder who seek therapists skilled in this modality. Even with the help of our many colleagues who are experienced SRT providers and trainers, there is no way we can possibly meet this need. Happily, this workbook brings SRT to all who wish to improve the stability of their social rhythms from the convenience of their homes; it extends the reach of SRT to many who will benefit from its techniques. With this beautifully written and exceptionally detailed explanation of what individuals with bipolar disorder can do on their own to achieve the more regular daily routines that are the core of SRT, self-directed treatment has become a possibility. For those fortunate enough to have a therapist who is already trained in social rhythm therapy or who is willing to learn along with you, this book provides an outstanding adjunct to treatment.

When training therapists in SRT, I often say that it's basically living life as your grandmother would have told you to live it. Wise grandmothers tell us to get up at the same time every day, eat regular meals, stay active, spend time regularly with those you care about, and get a good night's sleep. Now you can put your grandmother in your proverbial pocket and keep her with you all the time, guiding you to increased mood stability, better general health, and more enjoyment of your life.

—Ellen Frank, PhD
Professor of psychiatry and psychology, emerita,
University of Pittsburgh; Author of *Treating Bipolar Disorder: A Clinician's Guide to Interpersonal and Social Rhythm Therapy*

Introduction

If you seek new skills to better manage your bipolar disorder, this book is for you. Unlike most other self-help approaches, social rhythm therapy (SRT) focuses on the relationship between circadian rhythms (biologic processes that run on an approximately 24-hour schedule) and mood. Through a series of guided exercises, you'll learn to recognize and regularize your daily routines (social rhythms) with the goals of stabilizing circadian rhythms and improving mood. Following this research-proven approach to improving health, you'll acquire new and biologically informed strategies to gain better control over your bipolar disorder.

Why is this workbook unique? Abnormalities in circadian rhythms, or "biologic clocks," have been implicated in the onset and maintenance of bipolar disorders.[1] SRT consists of novel behavioral strategies to help individuals stabilize their biologic clocks, which in turn helps stabilize mood. SRT is the only circadian-focused therapy for bipolar disorders, and this workbook is the first to focus on this treatment.

What is social rhythm therapy? Interpersonal and social rhythm therapy (IPSRT) was developed and tested by Ellen Frank and colleagues at the University of Pittsburgh as a treatment for bipolar disorder.[2] IPSRT comprises two components: interpersonal psychotherapy, which targets problematic interpersonal relationships, and SRT, which targets biologic clocks.[3] SRT comprises a set of principles and strategies originally developed for IPSRT, a well-established therapy for bipolar disorder.[4] Over time, social rhythm elements were distilled from IPSRT and organized into a separate, free-standing treatment framework now known as SRT. This workbook is a self-guided version of SRT, the component of IPSRT that focuses on circadian rhythms.

What can I expect from this workbook? This workbook walks you through steps you can take to stabilize your circadian rhythms by developing more regular routines. Each chapter provides information about biologic clocks, bipolar disorder, and social routines. Chapters also include exercises to better understand and then modify your daily rhythms. You'll learn how to use a self-assessment tool, the Social Rhythm Metric (SRM), to monitor and modify your social rhythms.[5] You'll be asked to rate your mood and track your social rhythms daily. Copies of the SRM can be found in the appendix and on New Harbinger's website for this book: http://www.newharbinger.com/51246. As you develop more regular routines, your mood will improve.

How to use this book.

- Aim to complete one chapter per week. Each chapter is conceptualized as a weekly lesson. Week-long pauses between chapters give you time to collect information about your routines on the SRM and therefore a clearer idea of changes you wish to make. Reviewing your SRM weekly will provide you with useful information as you advance through the chapters.

- Work at your own pace. Although the book is envisioned as eleven weekly lessons, you should decide what pace works best for you. Some individuals will be eager to forge ahead, reading the entire workbook over a short period of time. Others might need to take more time working through the exercises. In the end, you'll find your own rhythms (pun intended!) for moving through the book.

- Use this workbook by yourself or with a therapist. Although designed as a stand-alone workbook, you may wish to share the results of your social rhythm monitoring and goal setting with your therapist or doctor so they can support you in your work toward attaining regular rhythms. Therapists may choose to supplement individual or group therapy, assigning between-session activities and exercises from the workbook.

- Plan to complete the SRM daily. While working on your social rhythms, you should complete your SRM daily, beginning with chapter 2. Daily monitoring will help you get the most out of this workbook. Of course, many people struggle with daily monitoring. This workbook includes plenty of tips if you have difficulty completing your SRMs (see chapter 4).

Behavior change is hard. If you ever tried to lose weight or stop smoking, you know that behavior change is rarely easy. The process of changing your social rhythms, like any habit, can be hard. In this workbook, you'll be encouraged to set goals for yourself. As you move through the workbook, push yourself to change your social rhythms but also be kind to yourself if you falter. Improvement rarely moves in a straight line; give yourself permission to take a few detours on your path toward social rhythm regularity and mood stability.

CHAPTER 1

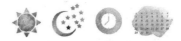

What Are Circadian Rhythms and Body Clocks?

Have you ever noticed that you're sleepy when you should be alert? Or wide awake when it's time to sleep? Do you get hungry outside of regular mealtimes? Does your energy level lag in the morning and pick up later in the day? If you have bipolar disorder, you have probably struggled with most, if not all, of these issues. Problems with sleep, energy, mood, appetite, and activity are core features of bipolar disorder; they are also greatly affected by circadian rhythms and body clocks. Circadian rhythms are patterned, physiologic activities and behaviors that run on an approximately 24-hour schedule, for example the sleep-wake cycle. Circadian rhythms and the body clocks that control them will be explained in detail in this chapter.

If you have bipolar disorder, you have differences in your biology that make you more likely to have unstable circadian rhythms and body clocks.[6] Abnormalities in circadian rhythms may underlie the development of mood disorders, such as bipolar disorder. When your circadian rhythms are unstable, your mood is worse. Interestingly, some medications used to treat bipolar disorder may work by improving circadian stability.[7] Behavioral strategies can also help to stabilize body clocks, thereby helping you feel better.[8] When your body clock and circadian rhythms are stable, your mood will be more stable too.[9]

This workbook focuses on helping individuals with bipolar disorder understand circadian rhythms and body clocks and learn skills to keep them running smoothly. These skills, known as social rhythm therapy (SRT), will help you feel better and stay well. Learning to manage your social rhythms and routines will help you to take control of your bipolar disorder.

In this chapter, we'll explore the science behind circadian rhythms and body clocks. We'll examine relationships between circadian rhythms and bipolar disorder. You may not be aware of them, but circadian rhythms have a big impact on your body and your mood. Learning more about circadian rhythms and body clocks is the first step in gaining better control of your body's rhythms and your bipolar symptoms.

What are body clocks? Body clocks are biologic processes involving genes, proteins, and hormones that keep circadian rhythms running smoothly, following an approximately 24-hour pattern across the day. If you have bipolar disorder, your body clocks are less regular than in someone without the illness.[10] Since many behaviors are affected by body clocks (e.g., sleeping, energy levels, eating), having bipolar disorder puts you at risk for having irregular patterns of sleep, energy, and hunger. Irregular body clocks and circadian rhythms are both a consequence of having bipolar disorder (i.e., your genes and biology predispose you to having irregular circadian rhythms) and a result of bipolar disorder mood shifts (i.e., bipolar mood episodes can themselves contribute to disturbances in circadian timing).[11]

Kylie has bipolar disorder. Her sleep schedule, energy level, and appetite are very different from her roommate Ally's. Ally, who doesn't have bipolar disorder, seems to effortlessly wake up at 6:30 a.m., work out for an hour, and arrive at work before 9 a.m. in good spirits. She is energetic and cheerful in the morning. She eats three meals daily, seems to have an even mood, and has a stable romantic relationship. Falling asleep by 11 p.m. each night is not a problem. Ally's biology makes it easy for her to stay on a regular schedule, helping her body clocks stay in sync with the external environment.

In contrast, Kylie is constantly "off schedule" or out of sync with her environment. Although she sets an alarm for 7 a.m., she often sleeps through her alarm or rolls over when it goes off because she is too tired to get up. She has been late for work so often that her job is in jeopardy. She is irritable and sluggish in the mornings, drinking coffee to stay awake. She can't concentrate well until early afternoon. Usually, she takes a nap as soon as she gets home from work instead of eating dinner. Her meals are "all over the place," at random times throughout the day. Although she knows she must get up at 7 a.m. to go to work the next day, she has a lot of trouble falling asleep before 1 a.m. She notices she is more energetic at night and doesn't feel like going to bed. She spends the evenings trying to catch up on household chores but often gets derailed by social media and video streaming. By 1 a.m., she forces herself to lie down although she often feels she could keep going for another few hours. Kylie's biology means that her natural body clock runs later than the clocks in her environment, likely related to having bipolar disorder. She constantly feels like she is "off schedule" relative to her work expectations and compared to friends like Ally. Being "off schedule" has a negative impact on her mood, life, and energy.

Disrupted body clocks lead to disturbances in sleep, energy, mood, appetite, and activity. Like Kylie, if your body clock is out of sync with external clocks, it can be difficult to get up for work on time, keep a household running, and maintain healthy relationships. Although it can be challenging at first, keeping body clocks in sync with external clocks is key to wellness for individuals with bipolar disorder. SRT helps you keep your body clock running smoothly by teaching you to establish and maintain regular daily routines.

What are rhythms? Rhythms are sounds, movements, or activities that follow strong, regular, and repeated patterns. Examples of rhythms include the bass line in a musical score, heart beats, and iambic pentameter in poetry. We also find rhythms in nature, such as the rising and setting of the sun, seasonal changes in plants, and ocean tides. We talk about the rhythm of life (birth, childhood, adolescence, middle age, old age, death) because it follows a fixed pattern. Routines of daily living such as childcare responsibilities or work schedules are also examples of repeated patterns that figure prominently in many lives. Rhythms are predictable because they follow an expected sequence, and we know what will happen next because we know what happened previously. When you have bipolar disorder, however, your biology may make some of your personal rhythms fall out of synchrony with the rhythms in the world around you. This mismatch between your internal rhythms and those of the external world contribute to worse moods and mood episodes.

By contrast, regular routines or social rhythms act as signposts for your body clock, helping it to know what to do or expect next. When you have bipolar disorder, you can modify your social rhythms to help your internal body clocks align with clocks in the outside world. That, in turn, will help improve your mood.

What do body clocks have to do with bipolar disorder? When you have bipolar disorder, it's harder for your body clock to stay regular.[12] It's much more sensitive to shifts in schedules, time zones, and routines.[13] Abnormalities in the circadian system have been found in individuals with bipolar disorder, both during well and ill periods.[14] These differences have been found using measurements of activity (actigraphy), sleep (polysomnography), and blood tests for hormones such as melatonin and cortisol.[15] When your body clock gets off track, it's harder for it to get back on track. When your body clock is off track, you feel worse.[16] Importantly, when you don't stick to regular daily routines, your body clock is easily confused, and your mood will worsen.[17]

EXERCISE 1.1 Noticing Rhythms

Rhythms can be found in nature and in our daily lives. Recognizing (and eventually reinforcing) naturally occurring rhythms in your life can help to stabilize your body clock. The more regular your daily rhythms, the more regular your body clocks. The more regular your body clocks, the more regular your moods.

What kind of rhythms or routines do you notice in your environment? Write examples of familiar rhythms in the space below (an example for each type of rhythm is provided to get you started!).

I notice these rhythms in *nature*:

tides at the shoreline; low tide in the morning and night and high tide midday

I notice these rhythms in *my own life*:

picking my kids up at the bus stop at 3:15 p.m.

What are circadian rhythms? Circadian rhythms are physiologic rhythms that run on an approximately 24-hour cycle. The word *circadian* comes from two Latin words, *circa*, which means "around" or "approximately," and *dies*, meaning "day".[18] This term was coined by Franz Halberg in the 1950s to describe bodily functions that fluctuate predictably over the course of a 24-hour period.[19] Examples of circadian rhythms in humans include the sleep-wake cycle, digestion patterns, and body temperature.

All living creatures, including plants, have circadian rhythms.[20] These rhythms have evolved over time to help life forms exist more harmoniously with their environment. Plants, for example, are less active during the night, when sunlight is absent, and more active during the day, when sunlight is plentiful. Leaves and petals unfurl during the day to facilitate photosynthesis and interact with pollinators but then retract as night falls.

Circadian rhythms run on an approximately 24-hour cycle. The word "approximately" is used to describe circadian rhythms—i.e., they run on approximately 24-hour cycles. In fact, normal human circadian rhythms are somewhat *longer* than twenty-four hours. Although all animals (and plants) have internal clocks that keep circadian rhythms on a 24-hour-plus cycle, biologic clocks drift without additional input from the outside environment. To keep circadian timing in sync with the 24-hour light-dark cycle, the circadian system uses feedback from external sources to constantly reset itself. This is helpful because the external environment is constantly changing (for example, longer days in the summer and shorter days in the winter); the interplay between the internal and external rhythms allows your body to stay harmonized with your environment.[21]

Information about *when* you are in the 24-hour cycle comes from many external factors including the angle of the sun relative to the horizon, the amount of light or dark in your environment, timing of exercise, whether you're upright or horizontal, and meals. Without this feedback, circadian rhythms would gradually drift forward in time, shifting by as much as an hour per week.

Circadian rhythms across the day. Circadian rhythms vary somewhat from person to person, with more variability in those with bipolar disorder. Factors such as age and having bipolar disorder affect the timing of your circadian rhythms.[22] Typically, individuals with bipolar disorder have later or delayed circadian rhythms compared to non-affected adults.[23] Adolescents have later or more delayed circadian rhythms compared to young children.[24]

Figure 1 depicts an example of circadian rhythms in an average adult human. Typically, melatonin levels (the sleep hormone) start to rise around 9 p.m., preparing our brains for sleep. As we fall asleep around 11 p.m., bodily functions, such as appetite and bowel movements, are suppressed. Body temperature and blood pressure decrease throughout the night. As morning approaches, melatonin levels drop. Concurrently, cortisol levels (an activating hormone), body temperature, and blood pressure rise, which in turn prepare the body for waking. During the early morning hours, bowel movements and hunger, which had been suppressed overnight, become more likely. Concentration and alertness, low during the night, are highest in the morning. Reaction times and gross motor function peak in the late afternoon, probably because our ancestors needed optimal muscle functioning at that time of day to catch prey.

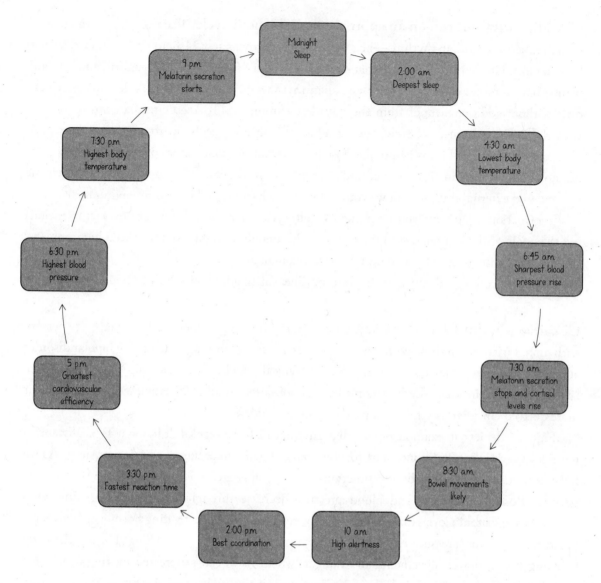

Figure 1. The Body's Rhythms Across Twenty-Four Hours

Although you may not have spent much time thinking about your circadian rhythms, you probably have noticed at least some of them:

- When you wake up, you may notice that you're hungry and have the urge to move your bowels or urinate. This is because digestion and elimination systems shut down at night so that your body can rest more easily; when you wake up, your digestive tract and elimination systems come back to life.

- If you wake up in the middle of the night, you may feel cold and want an extra blanket. This is because body temperature is lowest during sleep, which helps conserve energy.

- You get a better workout at 5 p.m. than at 8 a.m. This is because overall physical fitness increases in the late afternoon and early evening, which is when our ancestors would have been out hunting game.

EXERCISE 1.2 Janelle's Circadian Rhythms

Janelle uses SRT to stabilize her body clock. She is very aware of the effects of circadian rhythms on her body and behavior. Below, Janelle describes her daily rhythms. Underline examples of *actions* that Janelle takes to stabilize her circadian rhythms and circle examples that show the *effects of circadian rhythms* on Janelle. Examples are given in the first two lines.

I always set my alarm for 8 a.m., even on the weekends. I used to be groggy at 8 a.m., as if I were still asleep; I felt a strong urge to go back to sleep. But now that I am sticking to a regular wake-up time, I feel refreshed when my alarm goes off, as if my body clock realizes that it's time to be alert. I know that I'll have to use the restroom as soon as I wake up, which seems to be part of what happens when my body starts its day. I try to eat at least a small meal before leaving for work at 9 a.m. I don't really love eating breakfast but having something in my stomach helps me to feel more alert and have more energy in the mornings. It's been easier for me to focus and concentrate at work since I've been on this new schedule. I always have a dip in energy, however, after lunch. I often feel like I want to take a nap around 2 p.m., but I don't nap at work!

I'm naturally a night owl. Evenings are when I'm most energetic. I exercise right after work, usually around 6 p.m. to burn off some of that energy. I try not to exercise too late in the evening so that it doesn't keep me awake. By 7 p.m., I'm always hungry. I make sure I eat dinner before 8 p.m. so I'm not too full when bedtime approaches. Because it's sometimes hard for me to fall asleep by midnight, I start winding down for bed at 11 p.m. To get ready for sleep, I take a warm shower, turn off my screens, and read a book. If I follow my wind-down routine, I can usually fall asleep without too much difficulty.

Where is my body clock located? Body clocks are biologic pacemakers or internal clocks that keep physiology running on a 24-hour cycle. They comprise complex sets of genes and proteins that control many bodily functions.[25] The main body clock is in a part of the brain known as the suprachiasmatic nucleus, or SCN. Cells in the SCN "fire" on an approximately 24-hour cycle, producing many of the observed circadian rhythms in humans. The SCN is called the "master clock" and serves as the reset button and monitoring hub for the circadian system.[26]

The SCN is ideally situated to ensure that circadian rhythms generated by this pacemaker also respond to environmental cues: the SCN is found in the front part of your brain, close to your eyes. Specialized nerve pathways convey information about light and dark from your eyes directly to the SCN. Thus, the SCN can respond to changing environmental light conditions based on input received through your eyes. It's an elegant system: the body clock keeps its own time, but it can shift as needed when modified by external signals.

In addition to the SCN, there are body clocks located in virtually every organ of the body.[27] Body clocks in the liver and stomach affect digestion while clocks in blood vessels work with clocks in the heart to manage blood pressure.[28] These ancillary body clocks are in constant communication with the master clock, allowing synchronization of circadian rhythms throughout the body. When it's time to sleep, the SCN "tells" the hypothalamus to secrete melatonin (the sleep hormone again!), which in turn "tells" the other body clocks to regulate functions to accommodate sleep.

Information from peripheral (i.e., not located in the brain) body clocks is relayed back to the SCN. When you eat breakfast in the morning, the body clocks in your digestive tract send messages to the SCN effectively saying, "Our human is awake! It's eating food!".[29] The reciprocal inputs to and from ancillary body clocks help to keep circadian rhythms running smoothly.

You'll sense that your body clocks are working when you pay attention to how you feel and what you do at specific times of the day. For instance, you may notice you're hungrier at certain times rather than others. You might be aware (or become aware) of times of day when you're most energetic or best able to concentrate. You probably know when it's easiest for you to sleep (nighttime for most people, but not everyone). These behaviors are all evidence of working body clocks, or circadian rhythms.

EXERCISE 1.3 My Body Clock

Below is a personalized body clock and a list of common daily activities. Write the number of each activity on the clock face to indicate the approximate time that you're most likely to do it.

1. Wake up

2. Go to work or start daily chores

3. Feel most alert

4. Exercise

5. Get hungry or have meals

6. Concentrate on a project or on reading

7. Get sleepy

8. Go to bed

9. Fall asleep

10. Other (add your own personal activity): _____

This exercise will help you understand that many of your usual activities follow regular daily patterns.

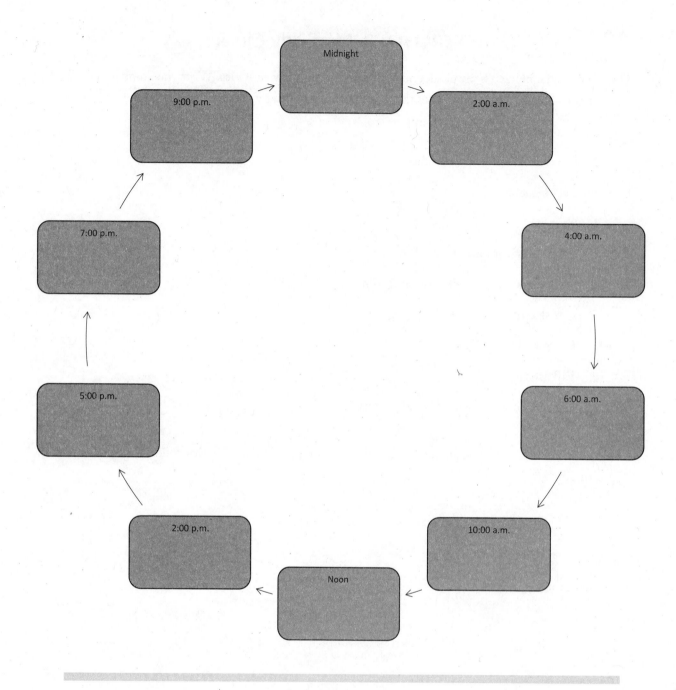

What keeps body clocks ticking regularly? In 2017, the Nobel Prize in Physiology or Medicine was awarded to Jeffrey C. Hall, Michael Rosbash, and Michael W. Young for their discovery of a gene that controls normal daily biologic rhythms.[30] They showed that the aptly named *period* gene controls the periodic expression of a protein, PER, that builds up in cells at night and degrades during the day. They also showed that cells have self-sustaining mechanisms, including an inhibitory feedback loop, that maintain expression and degradation of PER on a 24-hour cycle. In other words, circadian rhythms are hard-wired into our genetic material.

The Nobel laureates conducted their work in fruit flies, underscoring the ubiquity of these systems in nature. Research has also been done on circadian genes in mice. Mice that are genetically modified to lack some of these clock genes show behavioral patterns similar to mania: they sleep very little, engage in promiscuous (for mice) behaviors, and take more risks.[31] Interestingly, these behaviors can be reversed by lithium, a medication used to treat bipolar disorder.[32] Studies like these suggest that circadian clock genes may be affected in humans with bipolar disorder.[33]

What is a chronotype? Chronotype is the natural predisposition of your body to be more active or sleepy at certain times of the day.[34] Individual chronotypes include "larks" (a preference to be active in the mornings and a tendency to get sleepy relatively early in the evenings), "owls" (partiality for staying up late at night and tendency to have trouble waking up in the mornings), and intermediate types (neither larks nor owls). Chronotypes are often described on a spectrum of morningness (larks) and eveningness (owls), with a majority of individuals falling in the center of this spectrum (intermediate types).[35]

Chronotype is a behavioral manifestation of underlying circadian rhythms and appears to be genetically determined.[36] Biologically related individuals often share tendencies toward morningness or eveningness, thus chronotype is heritable. Age also affects chronotype[37], with very young children tending toward morningness, adolescents toward eveningness, and older adults moving back toward morningness. Many individuals with bipolar disorder have an evening (owl) chronotype.[38]

Is chronotype adjustable? Although chronotype is heritable and a relatively stable trait in adults, it can be affected by the environment. If you're naturally an owl but must get up every morning at 6 a.m. to care for small children, you may start to show a behavioral profile more characteristic of a lark-ish person. However, without the reinforcement of morning commitments, your schedule will very likely drift back toward your natural owl-ish schedule. Similarly, morning types can force themselves to stay up later if their environment demands it (homework, job, family obligations), but they will likely feel most energetic in the morning and perhaps not get enough sleep because they find it hard to sleep past their normal early wake-up time. It's possible—but hard—to fight biology. Bottom line: You'll feel your best if you can adopt a schedule that matches your chronotype.

EXERCISE 1.4 What Is Your Chronotype?

Some of us are "larks" (morning chronotype); some of us are "owls" (evening chronotype); most fall in between larks and owls (intermediate chronotype). Inspired by the Morningness-Eveningness Questionnaire[39] but significantly altered from the original, these questions will help you determine your chronotype.

1. If you were entirely free to plan your day (no obligations), what is your preferred wake-up time?

   5 5:00 a.m.–6:30 a.m. (05:00 h–06:30 h)

   4 6:30 a.m.–8:00 a.m. (06:30 h–08:00 h)

   3 8:00 a.m.–9:30 a.m. (08:00 h–09:30 h)

   2 9:30 a.m.–11:00 a.m. (09:30 h–11:00 h)

   1 11:00 a.m.–12 noon (11:00 h–12:00 h)

2. If you had no obligations the next day, what time would you go to sleep?

   5 8:00 p.m.–9:00 p.m. (20:00 h–21:00 h)

   4 9:00 p.m.–10:30 p.m. (21:00 h–22:30 h)

   3 10:30 p.m.–12:00 p.m. (22:30 h–00:00 h)

   2 12:00 a.m.–1:30 a.m. (00:00 h–01:30 h)

   1 1:30 a.m.–3:00 a.m. (01:30 h–03:00 h)

3. How easy is it for you to get up in the mornings?

   1 Very difficult

   2 Somewhat difficult

   3 Fairly easy

   4 Very easy

4. When you wake up in the morning, how alert do you feel?

   ☐1 Not at all alert

   ☐2 Slightly alert

   ☐3 Fairly alert

   ☐4 Very alert

5. If you wanted to exercise, what would be your preferred time of day to be very physically active?

   ☐6 8:00 a.m.–10:00 a.m. (08:00 h–10:00 h)

   ☐4 11:00 a.m.–1:00 p.m. (11:00 h–13:00 h)

   ☐2 3:00 p.m.–5:00 p.m. (15:00 h–17:00 h)

   ☐0 7:00 p.m.–9:00 p.m. (19:00 h–21:00 h)

6. Because of your professor's schedule, you're required to take an online exam for a class from 10 p.m.–11 p.m. (22 h–23h). How well do you think you would perform on the test?

   ☐1 Would do well—this is a good time for me to think

   ☐2 Would do reasonably—this is an okay time for me to think

   ☐3 Would find it difficult—this is hard time for me to think

   ☐4 Would find it very difficult—this is a very hard time for me to think

7. How easy or difficult is it for you to stay awake past 9 p.m. (21:00 h)?

   ☐4 Very difficult

   ☐3 Somewhat difficult

   ☐2 Fairly easy

   ☐1 Very easy

8. At what time of day do you feel your best (most alert, best mood)?

    5   5:00 a.m.–8:00 a.m. (05:00–08:00 h)

    4   8:00 a.m.–10:00 a.m. (08:00–10:00 h)

    3   10:00 a.m.–5:00 p.m. (10:00–17:00 h)

    2   5:00 p.m.–10:00 p.m. (17:00–22:00 h)

    1   10:00 p.m.–5:00 a.m. (22:00–05:00 h)

9. Would you describe yourself as a lark (morning person) or an owl (evening person)?

    6   Definitely a lark

    4   More a lark than an owl

    2   More an owl than a lark

    0   Definitely an owl

_____Total points for all nine questions

Interpreting the results. The sum of items gives a score ranging from 7 to 43. Scores of 16 and below suggest that you may be an "evening type"; scores of 32 and above suggest that you may be a "morning type"; scores between 17 and 31 suggest you may be an "intermediate type." If you're interested in learning more about your chronotype, you can visit the Center for Environmental Therapeutics (https://cet.org) to do some more self-assessments.

Circadian rhythms and bipolar disorders. Researchers have shown that aspects of circadian biology are different in individuals living with bipolar disorder, compared to those without it.[40] Those with bipolar disorder are more likely to have an evening chronotype, delayed sleep-wake phase, and lower levels and later timing of melatonin secretion. Abnormalities in some body clock genes are likely.[41] Not surprisingly, when you have bipolar disorder, your body clock is much more likely to be sensitive to shifts in schedules, time zones, and routines. It's hard for your body clock to stay regular, and when your body clock gets off track, it's hard to get back on track. Loss of regular routines is associated with worse mood, lower energy, disrupted sleep, and risk for mood episodes. Conversely, more regular routines are associated with improved mood, energy, and sleep, and less of a risk for new mood episodes.

Summary. Abnormalities in circadian rhythms seem to be both a cause of bipolar disorder and a product of the illness itself.[42] Developing regular daily routines to address disturbances in circadian rhythms is an important strategy to manage bipolar disorder.[43] SRT will help you learn how to regulate your body clocks, which in turn will help improve your bipolar symptoms and decrease your risk for a new mood episode.[44]

In the next chapter, we'll introduce the concept of social rhythms and start working with the Social Rhythm Metric, a self-management tool to help regulate social rhythms, body clocks, and circadian rhythms.[45]

CHAPTER 2

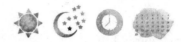

What Are Social Rhythms?

In this chapter, we'll discuss social rhythms. Social rhythms are interpersonal or socially regulated factors that affect circadian rhythms. Social rhythms are both a product of circadian rhythms (eating meals with friends when you feel hungry) and a driver of circadian rhythms (getting up at the same time every day because you have to go to your job). If you have bipolar disorder, having regular social rhythms can help improve your mood by stabilizing your circadian rhythms. In this chapter, we'll explore relationships among social rhythms, circadian rhythms, and mood.

What are zeitgebers? As discussed in chapter 1, body clocks depend on external cues to keep circadian rhythms running on a 24-hour cycle. These external inputs are known as zeitgebers. From the German word for "timekeeper," zeitgebers are rhythmically occurring environmental factors that entrain body clocks and circadian rhythms. You can think of zeitgebers as environmental anchors or signposts. Because of evolution and biology, the rising and setting of the sun is the most powerful signpost in our environment. Other important signposts include changing seasons, temperature, and food availability.

What is a social zeitgeber? When geophysical cues such as light are less pronounced, regular social interactions known as social zeitgebers or social signposts entrain the circadian system by acting as surrogate anchors or pacemakers. Examples of social signposts include work, meals, and leisure activities. Social signposts, therefore, are social factors that help our bodies keep track of time. Here are some examples of social signposts helping to entrain body clocks:

- *Tim's dog Bruno always wakens him at 6:30 a.m. to let him out. If Tim doesn't get up, Bruno whines and makes a mess in the house.* Bruno is a social zeitgeber or social anchor for Tim because he helps Tim get up at the same time every morning.

- *Even though they live far away from each other, Zenia calls her mother every day around dinner time. If she forgets to call, her mother gives Zenia a really hard time. Even though Zenia some-times resents having to call her mother, she almost never forgets that phone call.* Zenia's mother is a social zeitgeber for Zenia. Her phone call to her mother is a social signpost because it helps to mark Zenia's transition from daytime to evening.

- *Jeff's barista shift at a coffee shop starts at 7 a.m. To get to work on time, Jeff awakens at 6 a.m.* Jeff's work obligation acts as a social anchor for Jeff.

EXERCISE 2.1 Social Zeitgeber Checklist

Below is a list of common social zeitgebers, or things you might do around the same time every day to establish routines. Place a check mark (✓) next to any zeitgeber that applies to you. For items that you check, write in the time that you usually do the activity. See the example below. Write in any other social anchors that you can think of at the bottom. Only check the item if you do it *at about the same time almost every day*. Some of you might not have any regular anchors, especially if you have been depressed. That's okay, because this book will help you develop personal social sign-posts, which in turn will help keep your body clock on track.

☑ Feed the dog: 6:30 a.m.

☐ Eat breakfast: _____

☐ Eat lunch: _____

☐ Eat dinner: _____

☐ Go to school: _____

☐ Go to a work: _____

☐ Participate in _____
volunteer activity:

☐ Do housework: _____

☐ Walk my dog: _____

☐ Play a sport: _____

☐ Cook for my family:_____

☐ Attend organized _____
religious activities:

☐ Participate in _____
daily prayer:

☐ Exercise: _____

☐ Meditate: _____

☐ Take medications: _____

☐ Check my blood _____
sugar:

☐ _____

☐ _____

What are social rhythms? Do you get up when the sun rises and go to sleep when the sun sets? Probably not! In preindustrial, agricultural societies, circadian clocks were entrained almost exclusively by the rising and setting of the sun; in the modern world, however, we're no longer tightly bound to the natural environment. Consequently, our biologic clocks are at least partially entrained by recurrent social zeitgebers such as those that you identified in exercise 2.1. These repeating lifestyle or interpersonal routines that affect the biologic clock are known as social rhythms.

How do social rhythms affect mood? Regular social rhythms help to keep the body clock running smoothly. By doing the same thing at the same time every day, social rhythms remind the body clock *when* it is. Social rhythms help body clocks to stay on their roughly 24-hour cycle, thereby stabilizing circadian rhythms. If you have bipolar disorder, stable social rhythms will help your mood become or stay stable. The converse is also true, however: disrupted or irregular social rhythms may destabilize your circadian rhythms and make your mood worse. Therefore, the goal of SRT is to help you stabilize your social rhythms to stabilize your mood.

EXERCISE 2.2 Maria's Social Rhythms

Read Maria's story below to identify which of her social rhythms are regular, contributing to body clock regularity, and which are irregular and may get her body clock off track. "Regular" means that Maria does the same thing at almost the same time every day. "Irregular" means that Maria does not have a regular time for this activity. Examples of irregular rhythms are activities that are done at different times each day or are done on some days but not others. Irregular rhythms can also be the result of a major life change, such as having a new baby or new job.

Maria recently lost her job. Her mood has been worse both because she is unemployed and because her schedule is very different now that she is not working. She tries, however, to get up at the same time every day and find an activity to get herself out of her apartment. She sets up at least one meeting every day. Sometimes the meetings are to network for jobs. Other meetings are just to meet a friend for a walk or cup of coffee. Her finances are really tight, so she often skips lunch but she always tries to get some exercise, even if it's just a walk around the block. And, of course, she always calls her friend Angela to update her on her day. She knows that regular meals are important, so—although she skips lunch—she always makes herself something hot for dinner, even if it's just ramen noodles or rice and beans. She often has trouble falling asleep at night. Sometimes she watches videos on her computer until she can't keep her eyes open any longer. She often takes a warm bath before bed, hoping it will help her fall asleep.

Check boxes that apply to Maria and her routines.

Social Rhythm	Regular	Irregular
Work schedule		
Getting up at the same time every day		
Setting up at least one meeting every day		
Eating lunch		
Eating a hot dinner		
Talking to Angela		
Bedtime wind-down activities		

Social rhythms and bipolar disorder. Research has found that social stresses contribute to the onset of mood episodes and worsening of symptoms in bipolar disorder.[46] However, social stresses related to destabilized social routines or rhythms appear to be especially potent risk factors for worse outcomes in bipolar disorder.[47] Examples of social rhythm disruptions that put you at risk for mood symptoms include spending the night in the emergency room, staying up all night to study for an exam, or going on vacation. Disrupted or irregular social rhythms may lead to or be the result of a bipolar mood episode.[48] By contrast, periods of mood stability are associated with very regular social rhythms.[49] For instance, going to bed at the same time every day, eating meals at regular times, and exercising at the same time every day may help your mood. Having stable moods may also make it easier to stay on a regular schedule.

EXERCISE 2.3 Your Social Rhythm Regularity

Which of your social rhythms are regular? Which are irregular? Below is a list of common social rhythms. Check whether these social rhythms are regular or irregular in your life (you can also check that the rhythm does not apply to you). Write in additional social rhythms at the bottom. As a reminder, "regular" means that you do this activity at almost the same time almost every day. "Irregular" means you do not have a regular time for this activity or that you skip this activity some days. Thinking about your social rhythm regularity or irregularity will help you start thinking about rhythms that you want to stabilize.

Social Rhythm	Regular	Irregular	Does Not Apply
Time out of bed			
Work/job			
Daily housework			
Childcare responsibilities			
Eldercare responsibilities			
Petcare responsibilities			
Exercise			
Contact with another person			
Spiritual practice			
Breakfast			
Lunch			
Dinner			
Bedtime wind-down routines			
Time to bed			

EXERCISE 2.4 Remembering a Well Period

The goal of this exercise is to think about your routines and social rhythms during a well period—i.e., a stretch of weeks or months when your mood and energy were even or "normal," and you were able to function relatively well. If you're feeling that way now, reflect on your routines over the last few days. If you have been struggling recently, try to think back to a time when you were feeling well or stable.

Sleep schedule

Was your sleep schedule regular (i.e., getting up and going to bed at the same time every day)?   _____

On average, what time did you get up in the morning?   _____

On average, what time did you go to sleep at night?   _____

Were you napping regularly?   _____

How many total hours of sleep were you getting?   _____

Meals

Did you regularly eat breakfast? If so, at what time?   _____

Did you regularly eat lunch? If so, at what time?   _____

Did you regularly eat dinner? If so, at what time?   _____

Daily activities

Did you have a regular job or school during this time? If so, what and when?

_____

_____

Did you exercise regularly? If so, what and when?

_____

_____

Did you engage in any regular leisure activities? If so, what and when?

_____

_____

Did you engage in self-care activities? If so, what and when?

_____

_____

Personal connections

Did you have regular, daily contact with anyone? If so, with whom and when?

_____

_____

Did anyone help you stay on track with your routines (parents, partner, pets)? If so, who and how?

_____

_____

Did you have responsibility for others (children, parents, pets) during this time? If so, for whom and when?

_____

_____

After answering these questions, what do you conclude about the regularity (or irregularity) of your routines during this well period?

_____

_____

_____

EXERCISE 2.5 Remembering an Ill Period

The goal of this exercise is to think about your routines and social rhythms during a period of ill-ness—i.e., a stretch of weeks or months when your mood and energy were either high or low and you had trouble functioning. If you're having a hard time right now, reflect on your routines over the last few days. If you're feeling good right now, think back to your most recent mood episode or your worst mood episode and reflect on your routines at that time.

Sleep schedule

Was your sleep schedule regular (i.e., getting up and going to bed at the same time every day)?   _____

On average, what time did you get up in the morning?   _____

On average, what time did you go to sleep at night?   _____

Were you napping regularly?   _____

How many total hours of sleep were you getting?   _____

Meals

Did you regularly eat breakfast? If so, at what time?   _____

Did you regularly eat lunch? If so, at what time?   _____

Did you regularly eat dinner? If so, at what time?   _____

Did you have a regular job or school during this time? If so, what and when?

_____

_____

Did you exercise regularly? If so, what and when?

_____

_____

Did you engage in any regular leisure activities? If so, what and when?

_____

_____

Did you engage in self-care activities? If so, what and when?

_____

_____

Personal connections

Did you have regular, daily contact with anyone? If so, with whom and when?

_____

_____

Did anyone help you stay on track with your routines (parents, partner, pets)? If so, who and how?

_____

_____

Did you have responsibility for others (children, parents, pets) during this time? If so, for whom and when?

_____

_____

Reflections on exercises 2.4 and 2.5

As you think back on *both the well and ill periods* in your life, do you notice any relationship between the stability of your mood and the stability of your routines? If so, what did you notice?

_____

_____

If you noticed a link between instability of routines and your ill period, do you remember which came first? What happened?

_____

_____

Which types of routines (sleep, meals, daily activities, personal connections) seemed to vary the most between well and ill periods?

_____

_____

Introducing the Social Rhythm Metric (SRM). The Social Rhythm Metric, or SRM, is a self-monitoring tool that allows you to keep track of your daily routines and rhythms.[50] It takes less than two minutes to complete and should be filled out daily. Copies can be found in the appendix and on the New Harbinger website for this book, http://www.newharbinger.com/51246. The SRM allows you to see the relationship between your social rhythms and your mood. It will also allow you to set goals for your social rhythm regularity. You'll be completing the SRM daily while participating in SRT.

The SRM started out by tracking seventeen different daily routines.[51] However, researchers found that five specific daily activities were most strongly associated with outcomes in bipolar disorder. This version of the SRM therefore tracks only five daily routines.[52] These activities are:

1. Time out of bed

2. First contact with another person

3. Time starting usual daily activity

4. Dinner time

5. Bedtime

We added spaces in the SRM for you to add two regular activities that are personally meaningful, such as exercise, meditation, self-care, prayer, taking medication, and so forth. It's also okay to leave those extra activities blank since they were not part of the original SRM.[53]

SRM tips. Here are some tips about questions that commonly arise when completing the SRM.

Time out of bed

- Record the time that your feet hit the ground in the morning (your body clock has sensors that can tell you're vertical).

- If you're out of bed for at least thirty minutes, count that as your "time out of bed" (even if you go back to bed later for a nap).

- If you're awake but lying in bed, don't record "out of bed" until your feet are on the floor for at least thirty minutes.

First contact with another person

- This refers to your first reciprocal contact with another person. "Reciprocal" means that the other person responds to you in real time. Texts or instant messages count only if the other person responds immediately, as if you are having an in-person conversation.

- If you pass your roommate in the bathroom and they say hi, that counts.

- If your cat jumps on your head and wakes you up, that does not count. It must be a human.

Time starting usual daily activity

- Usual daily activity can be anything: a job, housework, classes, volunteer work. The idea is to pick something that you do several times a week.

- If you have different kinds of activities that you do during the week that get you moving, you can use a different activity for each day (for instance, on Mondays and Wednesdays, you watch your grandchildren, on Tuesdays and Thursdays, you volunteer in the local school, on Fridays you have a book club, and on Sundays you go to church).

- If you have no activity on a given day, you'll leave this field blank.

Dinner time

- Record the time that you eat (rather than prepare) dinner. Your body clock has sensors in the digestive tract that are affected by the time that you consume food.

- There are no rules about the size of the meal. A small snack counts.

- If you do not eat dinner on a specific day, leave it blank.

Bedtime

- Record the time that you turn out the lights for the night with the intent to go to sleep.

- If you're up and down multiple times during the night, record the time that you first tried to go to sleep for at least thirty minutes.

- If you fall asleep on the couch for an hour after dinner, get up, and then go to bed at 1 a.m. for the rest of the night, record 1 a.m. as your bedtime. The time on the couch would be considered a nap.

EXERCISE 2.6 SRM

Go to the New Harbinger website at http://www.newharbinger.com/51246 and print out a copy of the SRM (you'll need one SRM per week) or make copies of the SRM at the back of this book. Try filling out the SRM for the past twenty-four hours. If you're not sure what to record, reread the SRM tips above. Once you have completed one day's worth of information, you're ready to keep going, completing the SRM every day. It works best to pick a specific time of day to enter a day's worth of information. For instance, if you fill it out in the evening, complete the "bedtime" field for the night before and then enter the information for the current day except "bedtime," which you'll complete the following evening.

Leave the "target time" fields blank for now until you complete the exercise on SRM goal setting in chapter 4. It's helpful to complete at least a week of SRM information before starting to add in target times so that you get a feel for your current or baseline rhythms. There is also more information about rating mood and energy levels in the next chapter.

Summary. In this chapter, we identified routines that were associated with wellness (regular social schedules) and those that were associated with illness (variable or irregular social schedules). We also learned about the SRM, a tool that can help you keep track of your social rhythms, and ultimately help to stabilize them.

Since you already know a lot about body clocks, circadian rhythms, and social rhythms, you can start putting into practice some of the ideas discussed so far. For instance, complete this workbook at the same time every day to help anchor your daily routines. Or, you might think of another activity that you could try to do at the same time every day (e.g., have breakfast, exercise, meditate). Keep your goals small for now. Don't try to do too much at once but see if you notice differences in your mood by doing one or two activities at the same time every day.

In the next chapter, we'll look at bipolar disorder itself, learning about how doctors make a diagnosis and what symptoms are common to the illness. We'll also further explore the SRM, helping you to use this tool to notice patterns in your daily life that are associated with helping or destabilizing your mood.

CHAPTER 3

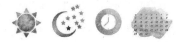

What Are Bipolar Disorders?

If you're reading this book, you have probably been told or believe that you have bipolar disorder. In this chapter, we'll take a closer look at bipolar disorder itself, learning about how doctors make a diagnosis and what symptoms are common to the illness. You'll learn that there are different kinds of bipolar disorder (type I and type II) and that doctors look for specific symptom clusters to determine a diagnosis. You may identify with some—but perhaps not all—of the illness descriptions. As you learn more about different kinds of experiences with bipolar disorder, you'll discover which symptoms are most relevant to you and therefore which ones to track over time as you work on stabilizing your routines. We'll conclude by discussing the SRM which was introduced at the end of chapter 2.

What are bipolar disorders? Previously called manic-depressive illness, bipolar disorders are a group of brain disorders that cause changes in mood and energy. There are several types of bipolar disorders, the most common being type I and type II (more about that soon).[54] Bipolar disorders are highly heritable, often running in families.[55] Bipolar disorders can start at any time in your life, but most commonly begin in early adulthood. Many individuals with bipolar disorder report that they had some symptoms in childhood, even if they did not experience "full blown" manic or depressive episodes.[56] Bipolar disorders are chronic conditions that wax and wane over time.[57] There are many treatments for bipolar disorders, including medications and psychotherapy.[58] SRT is a psychotherapy that has been shown to help improve outcomes for individuals with bipolar disorders.[59]

Bipolar disorders are defined by recurrent mood episodes, including depression, mania, and hypomania.[60] Hypomania—which is discussed below—is a less severe form of mania. When seeing a doctor for the first time, she will ask about your lifetime history of bipolar episodes (depression, mania, hypomania); she will make a diagnosis on the sum of your experiences over your lifetime rather than just your current mood state.

> *Anand recalls being depressed on and off "for as long as [he] can remember." He missed half of his tenth-grade classes because he was "so down [he] could barely get out of bed." He lost his appetite, had trouble concentrating, was filled with self-loathing, and slept ten to twelve hours per night. His family didn't believe in mental health treatment, so although his teachers urged his parents to take Anand to the doctor, he never went. By the spring of tenth grade, his mood had lifted. In eleventh grade, he began smoking a lot of marijuana, and he slacked off in school. He had hoped to go to a four-year college, but his grades from high school were not good enough. Instead, at age nineteen, he enrolled in a local community college to become a veterinary technician. His family refused to support him after age eighteen, so he also worked two janitorial jobs to pay for food, rent, and community college fees. He rarely had time to sleep because of all his commitments. Initially, he was tired all the time but soon his energy level "took off." His friends described him as "crazy hyper," and he was eventually hospitalized after breaking into a local library, allegedly to "learn everything in those books." When admitted to the hospital, he was told he was having a manic episode.*

Anand's doctor diagnosed him with bipolar I disorder because he had experienced a manic episode. To diagnose bipolar I disorder, all that is required is a single lifetime episode of mania.[61] Commonly, however, individuals with bipolar I disorder also experience episodes of depression. In retrospect, Anand probably had a depressive episode in high school (not diagnosed or treated) in addition to a manic episode at age nineteen. Thus, he would meet diagnostic criteria for bipolar I disorder with the typical pattern of experiencing both episodes of mania and major depressive episodes.

What is a major depressive episode? Many people think of bipolar disorder as "mood swings," but it really is much more than that. Mood may vary across the different phases of the disorder, but the episodes that define bipolar disorders comprise clusters of symptoms, of which mood is only one.

Requirements for a major depressive episode (this is the term that mental health professionals use to describe a "clinical" depressive episode) are codified in the World Health Organization's International Classification of Disorders (ICD). ICD is now on its eleventh edition (ICD-11).[62] According to ICD criteria, a depressive episode is defined as *at least* a two-week period of feeling sad, down, or uninterested in things. In addition, a clustering of symptoms (at least five of them) must accompany feelings of sadness including:

- Changes in appetite (eating too much or too little) with change in weight (gain or loss)

- Changes in sleep (sleeping too much or too little)

- Feeling sluggish or having low energy

- Observable agitation or psychomotor retardation (appearing to move slowly)

- Feeling bad about yourself, with low self-esteem

- Difficulty thinking clearly, focusing, or making decisions

- Feelings of hopelessness

- Feeling guilty

- Thinking about death, wishing for death, or attempting suicide

In addition, these symptoms must cause trouble in daily life, making it difficult to function normally or well.

Have you had experiences like this in your lifetime? If so, you very likely have had at least one major depressive episode, which, if paired with a lifetime history of a manic or hypomanic episode, will lead to a bipolar disorder diagnosis.

Are you currently feeling low or depressed? There are widely used screening tools for major depressive episodes ("clinical depression") easily accessible on the internet, such as the nine-item Patient Health Questionnaire (PHQ-9).[63] These tools will tell you whether you're *likely* to be experiencing depressive episode. Other factors, such as anemia, thyroid problems, or trauma, may contribute to feeling down, so you need advice from a knowledgeable doctor to sort it out. Only a qualified health professional can make a formal psychiatric diagnosis. *If you believe you're currently experiencing a major depressive episode, please contact your doctor or another qualified mental health professional.*

Suicide risk. Suicidal thoughts or behaviors can occur during both depressive and manic episodes but are much more common during depression. Studies have shown that individuals living with mood disorders are at increased risk for suicide attempts and death by suicide. Individuals with bipolar disorder are at twenty-five times greater risk for suicide than the general population.[64] Because suicidal thoughts or behaviors are symptoms of the illness, they typically improve when mood improves—although they sometimes persist even after the episode resolves. Suicidal behaviors and plans are life threatening and require immediate medical attention.

If you or someone you know is having thoughts of death or suicide, please contact the National Suicide Prevention Lifeline by calling or texting 988 from any telephone in the US. You can also text the Depression and Bipolar Support Alliance at 741-741. If you need immediate assistance, call 911 (in the US) or go to the nearest emergency room.

What is a manic episode? At least one lifetime episode of mania is required to make a diagnosis of bipolar I disorder. Mania can be very severe, sometimes requiring hospitalization. It almost always causes problems with jobs and relationships. A manic episode is defined as at least a one-week period of feeling "too" happy or being very irritable *and* having too much energy.[65] There is no upper limit on how long manic episodes can last. In principle, mania can last for weeks or months. Because mania is considered a psychiatric emergency, however, most individuals will receive medical treatment relatively quickly to manage the mania. As with a major depressive episode, a clustering of additional symptoms must accompany feelings of elevated or irritable mood to qualify for a manic episode, including at least several of the following:

- Feeling unusually good about yourself, like you're better than others

- Not needing very much sleep; feeling refreshed after just a few hours of sleep

- Talking a lot, going from topic to topic, so much so that others notice

- Finding that your attention is drawn too easily to unimportant factors in the environment

- An increase in sex drive, sociability, or goal-directed activities, such as cleaning, exercising, or work projects

- Engaging in dangerous or impulsive activities, such as spending a lot of money, driving dangerously fast, or impulsive recklessness without regard to the potential for negative consequences

- Unrealistic thoughts, like hearing voices that do not exist or feeling frightened for no reason

In addition, these symptoms must cause trouble in daily life, making it difficult to function normally or well.

Elenora reported a three-week period of elation before she went into the hospital in 2019. Although she had recently been let go from her job as graphic designer, she said that her mood was very good, and she felt on top of the world. She also had high energy throughout that time. She began collecting twigs, leaves, and dead insects in her basement to prepare for an "artistic project" that she thought had the potential to win her a Nobel Prize. Her roommates at the time kept asking her why she was collecting so much "junk," noting concerns that it might cause an insect infestation in their house. She reported that she became "snappy" with her roommates when they questioned her "important" activities. She also engaged in unusual behaviors such applying to join the Marines (she had no prior interest in the military) and going shopping for items she could not afford, such as a $500 comforter and a new iPhone. She began chatting *online with people whom she did not know in Brazil, her mother's home country. She made plans to travel to Brazil to visit these individuals, buying a business class ticket to São Paolo that she couldn't afford. She said that her sleep was reduced to two to three hours per night, but it didn't bother her because she felt "great." She began to act bizarrely, running out into traffic partially clothed, yelling in Portuguese. She was picked up by the police and admitted to a psychiatric hospital because of concerns about her erratic behavior and safety. The doctors told her she was having a manic episode.*

If you or someone you know is experiencing a manic episode, please contact your doctor or go to the nearest emergency room.

What is a hypomanic episode? Many people get confused about the difference between a manic and a hypomanic episode. "Hypo" means "below" in Greek. Hypomania is a lesser form of mania. Whereas mania can be very severe, often requiring hospitalization, hypomania never results in hospitalization and does not cause significant impairment in day-to-day functioning. In fact, some people feel like they are functioning *better* than usual when hypomanic. Hypomania can feel great for a while, but it doesn't last. Hypomanic episodes are not the same as feeling good for a few hours because you had some good news; it's a medical condition that lasts *at least several days* and can be recognized by others as a change from baseline. There is no upper limit on how long it can last. For some individuals, hypomania lasts for weeks or even months.

According to ICD-11,[66] a hypomanic episode is defined as at least several days of abnormally elevated or irritable mood and persistently increased activity or energy. As with a major depressive episode, a clustering of additional symptoms must accompany feelings of elevated or irritable mood including at least several of the following:

- Feeling unusually good about yourself, like you're better than others

- Not needing very much sleep; feeling refreshed after just a few hours of sleep

- Talking a lot, jumping from topic to topic, so much so that others notice

- Finding that your attention is drawn too easily to unimportant factors in the environment

- An increase in sex drive, sociability, or goal directed activities, such as cleaning, exercising, or work projects

- Engaging in dangerous or impulsive activities, such as spending a lot of money, driving dangerously fast, or impulsive recklessness without regard to the potential for negative consequences

In addition, these symptoms *cannot* cause psychosis (losing touch with reality) or make it difficult to function normally.

When Elenora was admitted to the hospital in 2019 for mania, her doctors asked her if she had had any episodes in the past like the current manic episode. She did not remember anything this extreme but recalled that, before she started her graphic design job in 2018, she had a weeklong period when her mood was very good, and she had high energy. She attributed it to being happy that she got a good job. But, like the beginning of the manic episode, she had been engaged in many activities and working out more than usual. Her sleep had been reduced to six hours a night, and she wasn't tired. She had gone out a lot with friends and spent more money on socializing than she should have. She hadn't been concerned, however, because she figured she could cover it when she got her first paycheck. Her friends thought then that she was "hyper" and talking fast. She had noticed that her libido was up, and she had hooked up with a few women whom she hardly knew. In retrospect, she noted that she didn't typically do things like that but "it was fun." When she started her new job, these experiences subsided. She went back to her usual level of activity and sleep. She didn't think it was a big deal at the time. The doctors told her that this was probably a hypomanic episode related to her bipolar disorder. They also pointed out that not having a regular schedule might have made her vulnerable to hypomania, which improved when she started the new job and got on a regular schedule.

What is the difference between a manic and hypomanic episode? Did you notice that the ICD-11 criteria for mania and hypomania are almost identical? This is the source of a lot of confusion! The key differences are:

- *Duration.* Mania must last at least one week (any duration if shortened by treatment) and hypomania must last at least several days. There is no upper limit on duration—i.e., both manic and hypomanic episodes can last for weeks or even months. Thus, if the episode has been going on for a few weeks, duration doesn't help distinguish the two episode types.

- *Functioning.* By definition, mania causes impairment in all areas of functioning but hypomania does not. In practice, this is a very thin line and can be hard to sort out.

- *Psychosis.* Psychosis may be present in mania but cannot be present in hypomania.

Why should you care if one of your "up" periods would be categorized as mania or hypomania? The presence of mania (versus only hypomania) leads doctors to make a diagnosis of bipolar I disorder. If *only* hypomania is present, a diagnosis of bipolar disorder type II (bipolar II disorder) would be given. Doctors treat bipolar I and II disorder differently, so it is important to make this distinction.

Although only a doctor can make a diagnosis of a manic or hypomanic episode, you can screen yourself for mania and hypomania using widely available scales (search for them online), such as the Altman Self-Rating Mania Scale (ASRM)[67] or the Mood Disorders Questionnaire (MDQ).[68] Note that these scales do not distinguish between mania and hypomania.

Mixed episodes. To make matters even more complicated, many individuals with bipolar disorder experience mixed episodes. Mixed episodes occur when an individual meets all criteria for an episode of mania or depression plus some symptoms of opposite polarity. For example, someone might experience sadness, low energy, suicidal thoughts, poor concentration, and poor appetite (i.e., they would meet ICD-11 criteria for a major depressive episode) while simultaneously experiencing racing thoughts, feelings of being better than everyone else, and not needing much sleep. Mixed episodes are common and associated with higher risk for suicide.[69]

EXERCISE 3.1 Identifying My Mood Symptoms

Not everyone experiences the same symptoms during mood episodes. This exercise will help you identify your personal mood symptoms in the context of mood episodes. These are the symptoms you'll target with more regular routines.

To better identify your personal experiences with depression, mania, and hypomania, think about how you feel during these mood states. Which symptoms are typical for you? Which ones are problematic? In the following exercise, put a check mark (✓) next to symptoms that you experience during each mood episode type. Add a plus sign (+) next to the check mark if it's problematic or upsetting to you. Note that some symptoms (such as irritability or poor sleep) may occur in more than one episode type.

Symptom	Episode Type		
	Major Depression	Mania	Hypomania
Sad or down mood			
Feelings of despair or hopelessness			
Irritability			
Loss of interest in usually pleasurable activities			
Feeling sluggish or slowed down			
Feeling bad about yourself, low self-esteem			
Difficulty thinking clearly or focusing			
Thinking about or attempting suicide			
Poor appetite or weight loss			
Increased appetite or weight gain			
Increased sleep			
Poor sleep/difficulty sleeping			
Upbeat or elated mood			
Increased energy/feeling wired			
Not needing very much sleep			
Talking fast about a lot of different topics			
Thoughts going very fast			
Feeling unusually good about yourself, like you're better than others			
Finding that your attention is drawn too easily to unimportant factors in the environment			
Doing lots of activities "on overdrive," such as cleaning, exercising, or work projects			
Engaging in dangerous or impulsive activities, such as spending a lot of money on unnecessary clothing, driving dangerously fast, or drinking too much			

Can I have both depression and bipolar disorder? If you have bipolar disorder, depressive episodes are considered part of your bipolar disorder diagnosis. You can't have both major depressive disorder and bipolar disorder. Once you experience even a single episode of mania or hypomania, your diagnosis changes from major depressive disorder to bipolar disorder. This distinction is important because medications for bipolar disorders differ from those used to treat major depressive disorder. Having both depressive and manic episodes is common in bipolar disorder, and depressive episodes occur more frequently in bipolar disorder than manic or hypomanic episodes.

What kind of bipolar disorder do I have? There are several types of bipolar disorder:[70]

- Bipolar I disorder—characterized by alternating manic and (usually) depressive episodes. Hypomanic episodes are also commonly present.

- Bipolar II disorder—characterized by alternating hypomanic and depressive episodes. Manic episodes *cannot* be present.

- Other specified bipolar and related disorders—alternating mild hypomanic symptoms (less than a "full" hypomanic episode) and depressive episodes.

Based on this logic, even one lifetime episode of mania means that you would be diagnosed forever with bipolar I disorder. An episode of hypomania could mean that you qualify for a diagnosis of either bipolar I or II disorder, depending on whether you have ever experienced an episode of mania. If you have had an episode of major depressive disorder but have never had a manic or hypomanic episode, you would be diagnosed with major depressive disorder. If you have had ups and downs but haven't experienced enough symptoms for either a major depressive episode or a manic or hypomanic episode, you may be diagnosed with "other specified" bipolar disorder.

EXERCISE 3.2 Bipolar Disorders Calculator

The bipolar disorders calculator can help you figure out what type of bipolar disorder you *may* have. Note that this does not take the place of a formal diagnosis, which must be made by a qualified medical professional.

Check which type(s) of episodes you have had *over your entire lifetime*. Use the definitions in the earlier part of the chapter to determine whether you have ever met the "technical" criteria for each episode type.

Episode Type	Yes	No
Major depressive episode		
Manic episode		
Hypomanic episode		

Scoring the bipolar disorders calculator:

Responses			
Major Depressive Episode	Manic Episode	Hypomanic Episode	Probable Diagnosis
Y	Y	Y	Bipolar I disorder
Y	Y	N	Bipolar I disorder
Y	N	Y	Bipolar II disorder
Y	N	N	Major depressive disorder
N	Y	Y	Bipolar I disorder
N	Y	N	Bipolar I disorder
N	N	Y	Other specified bipolar disorder
N	N	N	No mood disorder

Maybe it's not bipolar disorder? Other mental health disorders can be confused with—and sometimes co-occur with—bipolar disorders. These disorders include anxiety disorders, borderline personality disorder, post-traumatic stress disorder, attention deficit hyperactivity disorder, and substance use disorders. Sometimes medical conditions such as thyroid problems, anemia, and seizure disorders produce symptoms that can be confused with bipolar disorders. It's important to consider other possible explanations for your distress. For these reasons, it's always important to consult with a health professional for a complete evaluation of symptoms.

Mood disorders and circadian rhythms. As we discussed in previous chapters, having bipolar disorder—either type I or II—puts individuals at risk for disturbances in circadian rhythms. The risk goes both ways: having bipolar disorder means that your circadian rhythms may be more vulnerable to becoming irregular and having irregular circadian rhythms can worsen bipolar symptoms.[71] Interestingly, having major depressive disorder also is associated with disrupted circadian rhythms.[72] If the bipolar disorders calculator suggests that you have major depressive disorder, you might also find it helpful to regularize your social rhythms to stabilize your circadian rhythms. Studies of SRT have shown that these techniques are helpful for both depression and bipolar disorders.[73] We'll help you develop more regular routines, schedules, and rhythms in the next part of this book.

EXERCISE 3.3 Mood Thermometer

Each day, as part of completing the SRM, you'll rate your mood and energy levels. This exercise will help you personalize your mood ratings by developing your own personalized mood thermometer.

Imagine a thermometer with a range of –5 at the bottom and +5 at the top. In this scheme, "0" signifies an even or level mood rating.

0 = very level mood

In real life, we all have mild ups and downs. "Normal" mood ratings range from +1 to –1:

+1 = a little bit upbeat (how you feel after getting some good news)

–1 = a little bit down (how you feel when you're having a bad day)

Moods in the range of +2 to –2 suggest that early signs of depression or mania are present but not yet out of control. Here are some examples of what these ratings mean:

+2 = really up, starting to feel like nothing can get you down

–2 = low interest, pulling away from people and not wanting to talk much

Ratings in the 5 to 3 range are used when mood episodes are getting out of control (i.e., a rating of +/–4) or are extremely problematic (i.e., a rating of +/–5).

For mania:

+5 = most manic you have ever felt (usually requires hospitalization)

+4 = mania getting out of control

+3 = others notice that you are hyper, talking fast

For depression:

–3 = sad much of the time

–4 = depression makes it hard to function

–5 = most depressed you have ever felt (often requires hospitalization or immediate medical attention)

However, each person will experience slightly different symptoms at each level on the mood thermometer:

- In preparation for completing the personalized mood thermometer, think about symptoms you personally experience at each level of mood severity. For example, at +3, you may notice that you have trouble concentrating, and at +4, you become irritable.

- For each of the mood ratings listed below, you should add descriptions of what that level feels like *for you*. Here are some examples of descriptions you might consider writing on the blank lines, but feel free to use your own, based on your experience:

Can't be quiet, in other people's business

My mind can't settle down

Doing too many things, completing nothing

Really happy, nothing gets to me

Snappy and mean

A little sad, thinking about how bad everything is

No interests, feeling like a lump

Can't think of good reasons to live, feel like giving up

Crying all the time

Mark this page so you can use your personalized mood thermometer to help you fill out mood ratings on the SRM. You can also print a copy to keep handy from New Harbinger's website for this book: http://www.newharbinger.com/51246.

MY PERSONALIZED MOOD THERMOMETER

+5 really high, most manic, hospitalized:

_____

+4 mania getting out of control:

_____

+3 others notice that you're hyper, talking fast:

_____

+2 revved up, better than "normal" mood:

_____

+1 little bit upbeat:

_____

0 even or level mood:

_____

−1 little bit down:

_____

−2 sad, low interest:

_____

−3 others notice that you're down:

_____

−4 depression makes it hard to function:

_____

−5 really low, most depressed, possibly hospitalized:

_____

Common questions about mood ratings.

Q: If I was upset about something that happened at work, would I rate my mood as –1?

A: It depends on how upset you were. If it was just a blip, –1 would be right. If you spent the whole day crying and feeling like you wanted to crawl into bed, you might go for –2. If you had passing suicidal thoughts without a plan to harm yourself, maybe it would be –3.

Q: When I get manic, I get more irritable than happy. How would I rate that?

A: That's very common. The plus side of the scale is used for an overly happy or overly irritated mood. Most people at +4 or a +5 have some degree of irritability. The plus sign may be misleading. These aren't necessarily positive states, although they may feel that way some of the time.

Q: So 0 is good?

A: With this scale, a 0 is a normal or even mood.

Q: I am used to using a different scale to rate my mood. Can I use it instead?

A: Although we typically use this rating scale for the SRM, you can rate your mood using any scale that works for you.

Why should I rate mood and energy separately? Sometimes mood and energy go in opposite directions.

- Have you ever felt a little sad or down (mood = –2) while also feeling agitated or hyper (energy = +2)?

- Have you ever felt really good or upbeat (mood = +2) but still had some trouble getting going (energy = –1)?

Having mood and energy going in opposite directions is characteristic of mixed mood states.[74] It's therefore helpful to track mood and energy separately to see whether they are moving in the same direction or different directions.

EXERCISE 3.4 Energy Thermometer

The energy thermometer works like the mood thermometer.

The energy thermometer proceeds from +5 to –5.

> +5 = the most energetic you have ever felt
>
> –5 = the most slowed down you have ever felt
>
> "Normal" energy ranges from +1 to –1.
>
> +1 = a little bit energetic (how you feel after a cup of coffee)
>
> –1 = a little bit slowed down (how you feel after not getting a good night's sleep)
>
> 0 = calm; very even energy level

Energy in the range of +2 or –2 suggests that early signs of depression or mania are present but not yet out of control.

Here are some examples of what the ratings mean:

> +5 = superhuman levels of energy; moving faster than everyone else
>
> +4 = very energized; can't sleep or sit still
>
> +3 = others notice that you are restless, excitable
>
> +2 = a little hyper, starting to feel agitated, like a motor is revving up
>
> –2 = slowed down, feeling like it takes effort to do things
>
> –3 = others notice that you're moving slowly
>
> –4 = takes effort to do even small things; limbs feel heavy
>
> –5 = can barely move; in bed all day

However, each person will experience slightly different symptoms at each level on the energy thermometer:

- In preparation for completing the personalized energy thermometer, think about the kinds of energy levels you *personally* experience at each level of mood severity. For example, at +3, you may notice that you're restless or more active than usual, and at +4, you can't sleep.

- For each of the energy ratings listed below, add descriptions of what that level feels like for you. Here are some examples of descriptions you might consider, but feel free to use your own ideas:

So hyper that people say I'm bouncing off the walls

Lots of projects and activities

Pacing the floors, can't rest

Moving fast, really zippy

A little more energetic than usual

Sluggish, slowed down

Pushing myself to move, limbs feel heavy

My limbs can't move, like I'm in cement

Spending every second in bed, can't do anything

Mark this page so you can use this personalized energy thermometer to guide you when you fill out the SRM. You can also find a downloadable, printable copy of this exercise at http://www.newhar binger.com/51246.

MY PERSONALIZED ENERGY THERMOMETER

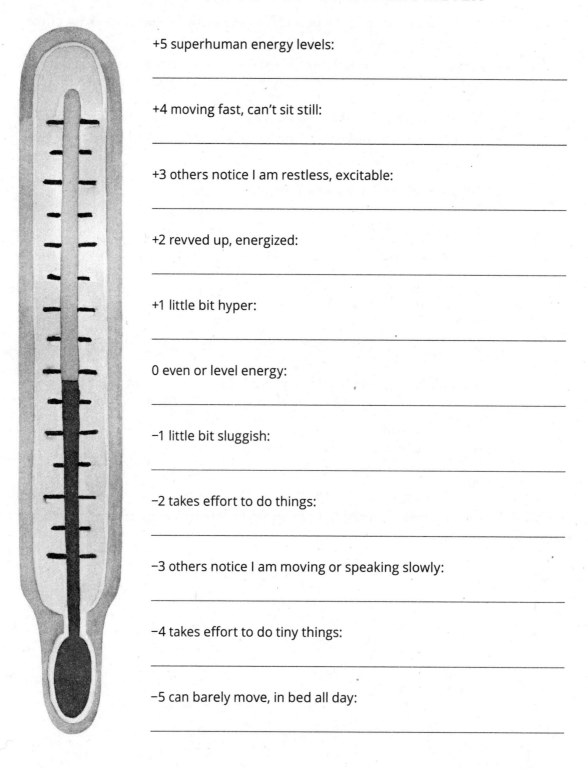

+5 superhuman energy levels:

_____

+4 moving fast, can't sit still:

_____

+3 others notice I am restless, excitable:

_____

+2 revved up, energized:

_____

+1 little bit hyper:

_____

0 even or level energy:

_____

−1 little bit sluggish:

_____

−2 takes effort to do things:

_____

−3 others notice I am moving or speaking slowly:

_____

−4 takes effort to do tiny things:

_____

−5 can barely move, in bed all day:

_____

Why include mood and energy ratings in the SRM? Inclusion of mood and energy ratings allows you see the links among your mood, energy, and daily routines. In SRT, we expect that your mood and energy will be worse when your schedules are less regular. As your routines become more regular, your mood and energy will improve.

Revisiting the SRM. While you're working on SRT, it's important to complete SRMs consistently to develop a fuller picture of your own social rhythms and their relationship to your mood and energy. If you're having trouble remembering to complete the SRM daily (a common problem, especially if you're not feeling well), we'll provide some tips and strategies in the next chapter to help you. If you have already completed *at least one week* of SRM monitoring, move on to the next chapter where you'll learn to analyze the SRM. If you're not ready for another chapter, continue to monitor using the SRM until you feel ready.

Summary. In this chapter, you learned about bipolar disorders. You're now familiar with symptoms that are commonly present in depressive, manic, and hypomanic episodes. You identified mood symptoms that are typical for you. As you develop more stable routines, we expect these symptoms to improve. If your symptoms are already improving, stability of routines will help keep them from getting worse.

In the next chapter, you'll learn how to analyze the SRM and discover strategies to help you overcome barriers to completing it.

CHAPTER 4

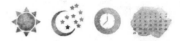

Using the Social Rhythm Metric

In this chapter, you'll learn how to use the Social Rhythm Metric (SRM) to track your daily rhythms and moods. You'll focus on analyzing information generated when you complete your SRM. This process will help you see the connections between rhythm regularity and your mood and energy. Although you won't be asked to change your routines (yet!), it will pave the way for modifying your routines in the following chapters.

Those of you who are in the "look before you leap" category will probably find it helpful to understand your routines before changing them, whereas the "eager beavers" may feel some frustration about having to wade through another chapter before getting tips on how to make changes (hang in there—soon!). Still others may find discovering how your irregular routines may have exacerbated your bipolar disorder an unsettling process. Taking a stepwise approach to this process (learning to analyze SRMs before modifying your rhythms) will help you feel ready to make the changes needed to help you feel better. If you start to feel overwhelmed, there will be tips throughout this chapter to make the change process more manageable.

In this chapter, you'll be asked to look at and evaluate your own SRM, so it's helpful to have completed at least one week of self-monitoring before proceeding. If you're having trouble completing your SRM, this chapter will also discuss strategies to address barriers to SRM completion. If you're not ready to analyze your own SRM, you can practice by analyzing the example provided (see "Caleb's SRM" later in this chapter).

The Social Rhythm Metric revisited. In this chapter, you'll learn how to analyze your SRM to see patterns in your routines. You should pay particular attention to which activities you do at (almost) the same time every day and which activities are less consistent. You should examine connections between consistency of your daily rhythms and your mood and energy ratings. Hopefully, you'll start to notice patterns that are either beneficial to or problematic for your mood and energy. These patterns will set the stage for learning in chapter 5 to set SRM target times and in chapter 6 to develop goals to improve rhythm stability.

This chapter will focus on understanding rather than changing your social rhythms. An analogy might be reading a cake recipe before starting to cook. It's important to know in advance how many eggs you'll need, whether to use one or two mixing bowls, how much flour to measure out, and at what temperature to preheat the oven. You could, of course, just improvise a cake recipe, but the final product usually comes out better if you follow the directions stepwise. Similarly, becoming familiar with your routines (which are regular, which are more irregular, how can you track your mood) will lead you toward a more reasoned and informed change process for your circadian rhythms. You need to know what's going on with your body clocks before you modify them.

Identifying and solving SRM monitoring challenges. If you're struggling to fill out your SRM daily, you're not alone. Many people have trouble filling out the SRM every day, especially if they're not feeling well. You might also imagine that completing the form will make you feel worse because you'll see in black and white how you're oversleeping or skipping meals or just feeling lousy. Part of you wants to close this book and never look at it again. And yet, as bad as it feels right now, part of you is looking for a change because you have already made it to chapter 4. Knowing that you might have mixed feelings about all this, I would encourage you to imagine what it might feel like to be less depressed, have more energy, and get your sleep back on track. Change is possible! Completing the SRM is an important tool for you to take control of bipolar disorder and enhance wellness. It will help you get to where you want to go. You don't have to do this on your own; this book will help you. The next exercise will help problem solve barriers to regular SRM completion.

EXERCISE 4.1 Barriers and Solutions to SRM Completion

Below is a list of common barriers to SRM completion. Check all that apply to you. In the space provided, brainstorm ideas on overcoming the barrier. If you can't think of any solutions, don't worry about it; there are suggestions for managing barriers at the end of the exercise. If you would like to repeat this exercise or have a hard copy for reference, you can find a printable copy of it on the website for this book: http://www.newharbinger.com/51246.

☐ I can't remember to complete my SRM every day: _____

_____

☐ I keep misplacing my SRM. I can't find it when I need it: _____

_____

☐ I don't have enough energy or motivation to complete it: _____

_____

☐ I avoid looking at my SRM because my life is such a mess: _____

_____

☐ I keep forgetting to enter my "time to bed": _____

_____

☐ I hate filling out paper forms: _____

_____

☐ Some of the items don't apply to me: _____

_____

☐ I'm good; I don't have any trouble completing my SRM daily: _____

_____

Here are some tips to help overcome common SRM completion challenges. Check the ones that might be helpful for you.

☐ Set an SRM reminder for yourself each day on your phone or computer.

☐ Fill out your SRM at the same time every day.

☐ Put your SRM somewhere that you're likely to see it every day, like taped to the bathroom mirror or on your bedside table. Keep a pen nearby!

☐ Filling out one or two items on the SRM is better than not tracking any items. Pick just one item to track this week.

☐ Record your "best guess" for your upcoming bedtime. If you end up going to bed earlier or later than expected, correct it the next day.

☐ If you didn't do an activity or can't remember, leave it blank.

☐ Be gentle with yourself if this is hard. Just do one item a day, taking it one day at a time.

☐ Create a spreadsheet on your computer and track your SRM information there rather than on the form provided.

☐ Leave a sticky note for yourself reminding you of why you feel it's important to monitor your SRMs.

☐ Ask a friend or relative to help you remember with a reminder text or call.

☐ Find an SRM buddy. Fill out your SRMs together.

List two things that you'll do this week to stay on track with completing your SRMs.

1. I will _____

2. I will _____

Tips for analyzing SRMs. When approaching a completed SRM, you should focus on patterns of regularity or irregularity in daily activities and then examine mood and energy ratings. When first approaching the SRM, look *across the rows* rather than up and down at the columns. This will help you to get a sense of how regularly you're doing each activity across the week. Try to find patterns in your routines: Do you have steady routines during the week but more erratic ones on the weekend? Did something happen in the middle of the week that threw off your routines for the rest of the week? Did you have consistency in some routines but not others?

Next, look at mood and energy ratings for each day. Do you notice a connection between your routines and symptom ratings? Can you see in your SRM the effects of your routines on your mood and energy? Is there a lag or delay in the connection between your routines and moods (this is a common pattern)? What happens to your mood and energy ratings when your routines are consistent? What happens to them when your routines are inconsistent?

EXERCISE 4.2 Analyzing Caleb's SRM

Caleb has bipolar I disorder and is learning to monitor SRMs. Look at Caleb's SRM and then answer the questions that follow. This will give you practice analyzing someone else's SRM before trying it on your own.

> *Caleb is twenty-five years old, identifies as nonbinary, and uses they/them pronouns. They work as a teaching assistant at a local elementary school. They usually get to work around 7:30 a.m. to get organized, and classes start at 8 a.m. Despite feeling a little down, they make it to work every day. They tend to isolate and oversleep on the weekends. They find that exercise is a very important part of wellness, so they work out every day. They go to the gym on their way home from work during the week and lift weights at home on the weekends. They are hungry after working out, so they always eat dinner as soon as they get home. They also find that, in general, they have more energy at night and like to stay up late playing video games. Here is Caleb's SRM for the past week.*

CALEB'S SOCIAL RHYTHM METRIC (SRM) #1

Activity	Target Time	Sunday Time	Monday Time	Tuesday Time	Wednesday Time	Thursday Time	Friday Time	Saturday Time
Out of bed		11 a.m.	6:17 a.m.	6:10 a.m.	6:45 a.m.	6:05 a.m.	6:05 a.m.	10:15 a.m.
First contact with other person		Noon	7:30 a.m.	7:30 a.m.	7:30 a.m.	7:30 a.m.	7:30 a.m.	11 a.m.
Start work/school/volunteer/family care		———	8 a.m.	8 a.m.	8 a.m.	8 a.m.	8 a.m.	———
Dinner		7:15 p.m.	6:15 p.m.	6 p.m.	6:30 p.m.	6:10 p.m.	6:10 p.m.	7:00 p.m.
To bed		1:30 a.m.	9:30 p.m.	11:30 p.m.	9:30 p.m.	11 p.m.	1:30 a.m.	Midnight
Exercise		Noon	4:30 p.m.	4:30 p.m.	4:45 p.m.	4:15 p.m.	4:30 p.m.	11 a.m.
Rate MOOD each day from −5 to +5 −5 = very depressed +5 = very elated		1	−2	−1	−2	−1	2	−1
Rate ENERGY LEVEL each day −5 = very slowed, fatigued +5 = very energetic, active		2	−2	−2	−2	0	1	−1

Answer the following questions about Caleb's SRM.

1. Caleb's *most* consistent activity was: _____

2. For the most consistent activity, the earliest time that they
    did it this week was: _____

3. For Caleb's most consistent activity, the latest time that they
    did it this week was: _____

4. Subtract the answer for #2 from #3 to calculate the range of
    time over which Caleb completed this activity this week: _____

5. Their *least* consistent activity was: _____

6. For their least consistent activity, the earliest time that they
    did it this week was: _____

7. For their least consistent activity, the latest time that they
    did it this week was: _____

8. Subtract the answer for #6 from #7 to calculate the range of
    time over which Caleb completed this activity this week: _____

9. Their lowest mood rating was _____ on (day) _____

10. Their lowest energy rating was _____ on (day) _____

11. Their highest mood rating was _____ on (day) _____

12. Their highest energy rating was _____ on (day) _____

13. Here is what I noticed about the relationships among Caleb's SRM activities, mood, and
    energy ratings:

    _____

Here are some notable findings from Caleb's SRM:

- Caleb's wake-up time was consistent during the week (within a forty-minute window Monday through Friday) because they had to get to work, but it was inconsistent on the weekends (10:15 a.m. on Saturday and 11 a.m. on Sunday). A mismatch between weekday schedules and weekend schedules is common. However, Caleb really paid for oversleeping on Saturday and Sunday when Monday morning hit. Getting out of bed when their alarm went off on Monday, Tuesday, and Wednesday was very difficult. On Wednesday, they were almost late for work (getting up at 6:45 a.m. instead of 6:05 a.m.) because they were so tired. Their mood suffered too, with worse mood ratings at the beginning of the week as they tried to get back on track with schedules.

- Their time to bed was all over the place, ranging from 9:30 p.m. to 1:30 a.m. Naturally a night owl, they gravitate toward staying up late unless they are exhausted. For instance, on Friday night they ended up going out to a bar and drinking too much, which they later regretted. They didn't go to sleep until 1:30 a.m., which led them to sleep late on Saturday (until 10:15 a.m.), even though they had wanted to get up early to exercise. By Sunday, they were completely off their weekday schedule.

EXERCISE 4.3 Analyzing My SRM

Now that you have practiced analyzing an SRM using Caleb's example, try analyzing your own SRM (if you have completed one). Pay special attention to the regularity (consistency) of your routines and the relationship of regularity of schedules to your mood and energy ratings. A regular or consistent routine is something that you do *at almost the same time every day*. Ideally, you would do an activity at the exact same time every day, within a forty-five-minute window. However, the more regular, the better, so completing the activity within a one-hour window would be considered better than completing it within a four-hour window. If you'd like to repeat this exercise, you can find it at http://www.newharbinger.com/51246.

1. My *most* consistent activity was: _____

2. For my most consistent activity, the earliest time that I did it
   this week was: _____

3. For my most consistent activity, the latest time that I did it
   this week was: _____

4. Subtract the answer for #2 from #3 to calculate the range of
    time over which you completed this activity this week: _____

5. My *least* consistent activity was: _____

6. For my least consistent activity, the earliest time that I did it
    this week was: _____

7. For my least consistent activity, the latest time that I did it
    this week was: _____

8. Subtract the answer for #6 from #7 to calculate the range of
    time over which you completed this activity this week: _____

9. My lowest mood rating was _____ on (day) _____

10. My lowest energy rating was _____ on (day) _____

11. My highest mood rating was _____ on (day) _____

12. My highest energy rating was _____ on (day) _____

Write down observations about your SRM, including the relationships among your SRM activities, mood, and energy ratings:

_____

_____

_____

_____

Summary. In this chapter, you learned to identify barriers and solutions to SRM completion. You also learned how to analyze SRMs to detect relationships between your SRM activities and mood symptoms.

In the next chapter, you'll learn how to set social rhythm targets using the SRM. Setting targets will be an important step toward stabilizing rhythms and thereby improving and stabilizing your mood. As you continue SRT, be sure to complete your SRM every day so that you can recognize patterns in your own life.

CHAPTER 5

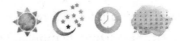

Setting Social Rhythm
Metric Targets

In this chapter, you'll be asked to look at your own SRM as you learn about setting target times, so you'll need to have your most recent SRM worksheet on hand. We'll also continue with Caleb's SRMs (introduced in chapter 4) to practice calculating and setting target times.

What does "regular" really mean? In this book, we talk a lot about regular routines and rhythms. But what, exactly, do we mean by "regular"? In research studies, the SRM defines an activity as "regular" if it occurs within a forty-five-minute window from day to day.[75] That means that an activity is considered regular if you do it within a forty-five-minute window of the target time (more on setting target times below). In community studies, most people do their daily activities within forty-five minutes of their usual or target time for that activity about half the days (three to four) of the week.[76] By contrast, individuals with bipolar disorder do their activities regularly on only two to three days per week. So *before* participating in SRT, individuals with bipolar disorder, on average, have fewer regular routines than those without bipolar disorder. However, *after* participating in SRT, individuals increase regular activities to five to six days per week. Although doing activities at the same time *every day* of the week remains the goal, even doing activities regularly five or six days a week was associated with better mood outcomes (lower risk of new mood episodes over a two-year period).[77] Research shows that the more regular your routines, the better your bipolar symptoms, including a lower risk of new mood episodes.[78]

What does this mean for you? Your goal will be eventually to complete most activities on your SRM within a forty-five-minute window of your target or habitual time, most days per week. That's a lot of regularity! We call these *supranormal* rhythms—i.e., routines that are even more regular than those of the general population.

What are supranormal rhythms? Supranormal means "above" normal or "more than" normal. If you have bipolar disorder, you should strive to have supranormal rhythms because it will help regulate your moods. In practice, this means being more regular with your routines than people without bipolar disorder. If your friend without bipolar disorder stays out late on Saturday night and then has trouble falling asleep on Sunday night, they can usually manage to recover on Monday, even after getting less sleep than usual on Sunday night. They may feel a little tired on Monday, but they quickly get back to their regular routines, and their mood remains stable. If you have bipolar disorder, however, getting off your routines on the weekend can be a big problem on Monday morning. Not only will you be sleepy on Monday, but your mood will also probably suffer. You may not have enough energy to eat dinner, which will further throw off your circadian rhythms. By Tuesday morning, instead of bouncing back, you may still feel down and have poor energy. Feeling down for a couple of days may lead to a depressive episode. It's much harder to rebound from schedule disruptions when you have bipolar disorder.

An analogy with diabetes is useful. Some of us are born with genetic predispositions to diabetes and others with genetic predispositions to bipolar disorder. Some of us have predispositions to both. Neither diabetes nor bipolar disorder is anyone's fault—and yet we can modify our behaviors to help us live more successfully with both these conditions. For instance, if you have diabetes, you must be extra careful about your sugar intake. To prevent your blood sugar levels from increasing, you need to eat fewer sugary foods than a person without diabetes. You will probably notice that eating sugary foods causes your blood sugar levels to skyrocket, making you feel sluggish and nauseated. If you have diabetes, you'll benefit from having extra-healthy (supranormal) eating habits. The same is true for schedules and bipolar disorder. Because your body clock is more sensitive than it is in someone without bipolar disorder, getting off a regular schedule confuses your body clock and makes you feel worse. By contrast, you'll feel better if you keep a very regular schedule—likely more regular than someone who does not have bipolar disorder.

Those with diabetes must eat less sugar to stay healthy, but people without diabetes also benefit from eating fewer sugary foods. Similarly having supranormal rhythms may also be beneficial to those without bipolar disorder. If you live with people who don't have bipolar disorder, they may wish to join you in your quest for rhythm regularity both as a show of support and because regular routines are probably good for everyone,[79] especially those at risk for cancer,[80] gastrointestinal diseases,[81] obesity,[82] HIV,[83] and heart disease.[84] If we think about all the people affected by these conditions, we can reasonably say that most of us—not just those with bipolar disorder—will benefit from regular routines.

What comes to mind when you think about supranormal rhythm regularity in your own life? Are you the kind of person who naturally gravitates toward regularity or do you hate feeling tied to a fixed schedule? Do you envision hurdles to developing supranormal routines? What do see as some possible benefits? Write down your reflections here:

Below is an example of someone who started SRT with trepidation. As you read about Angelina's experiences starting SRT, consider whether your reactions would be similar to or different from hers.

When Angelina started doing SRT, she was worried she would not be able to develop supranormal routines. She thought to herself, I like sleeping late on the weekends. All my friends sleep late on Saturday and Sunday, so why can't I? There is no way I am going to get up at the same time every day. She was also the kind of person who preferred spontaneity to predictability. The idea of following a regular schedule was frankly unpleasant. Because her mood was low, however, she was willing to try to adhere to more regular schedules to see if she felt better. Although initially resistant to the idea of getting up at the same time every day, including weekends, she reluctantly decided to try it out. She thought to herself, If this doesn't work, I can just go back to my usual routines. She was pleasantly surprised that after two weeks of getting up at almost the same time every day, her mood started to improve. She realized that supranormal routines helped her feel better. Angelina even convinced her roommate to get onto a regular schedule with her. Even though Angelina's roommate doesn't have bipolar disorder, they both felt better with consistent routines.

Are you like Angelina? Do you feel uncertain about making changes to your routines? If so, you're not alone. A lot of people feel some anxiety about trying to develop more regular routines. It may help to keep these ideas in mind: 1) You'll only make small changes at first, 2) If you don't like it, you can always stop, 3) If you don't try, you'll never know if it's helpful, and 4) It's okay to feel uncertain. Give yourself permission to be unsure about changing your routines but keep reading to learn more about how it *might* help.

Setting target times. *Math Warning!* The following section describes calculations used to set target times for each SRM activity, based on your current SRMs. You'll be asked to calculate averages, which means you'll have to add up all the numbers in a sequence and then divide by the number of items you added. It's not as bad as it sounds, but if doing math is too stressful for you, skip these calculations and make a guess about the average times you're doing each activity. The former strategy is more precise, but the latter strategy is okay too.

To calculate target times, first calculate the *average* time that you did the activity in the last one to two weeks, rounded to fifteen-minute increments. These calculations give you the midpoint of your circadian rhythms for each activity. You need to change hour/minute notations to numbers to do the math. For instance, 8:30 becomes 8.5 and 8:45 becomes 8.75. If your wake-up times for the past week were 7:30, 7:00, 9:30, 9:45, 7:30, 10, and 11:15, your target time would be 9 a.m. [(7.5 + 7 + 9.5 + 9.75 + 7.5 + 10 + 11.25) ÷ 7 = 8.9]. In this calculation, you would round 8.9 to 9, or 9:00 a.m. Divide by the total number of items you added.

This system works if all values are in the a.m. or all are in the p.m. If some of the values are in the a.m. and others in the p.m., however, you must convert to military time by adding twelve to the afternoon times. In military time, 10 a.m. is 10:00 h, 1 p.m. is 13:00 h, 2 p.m. is 14:00 h, and so forth. So, if your exercise times were 10 a.m., 11 a.m., 5 p.m., 4 p.m., and 4:30 p.m., you would use military time and divide by the number of times you did the activity [(10 + 11 + 17 + 16 + 16.5) ÷ 5 = 14.1, or 2 p.m.].

EXERCISE 5.1 Calculate Average Times

In this exercise, we'll revisit Caleb's SRM from chapter 4. For Caleb's SRM, calculate average times for each activity. We'll use this as a guide for setting Caleb's target times in the following exercise.

When calculating average times, round to the closest fifteen-minute increments. When Caleb lists 6:17 for their wake-up time, round it to 6:15 (6.25 for the purposes of doing the math). When they list 6:05, round to 6:00. Caleb's first activity is calculated for you.

Out of bed:

$$(11 + 6.25 + 6 + 6.75 + 6 + 6 + 10.25) \div 7 = 7:30 \text{ a.m.}$$

First contact with another person:

(_____ + _____ + _____ + _____ + _____ + _____ + _____ = _____) ÷ 7 = _____

Start work/school/volunteer work (Caleb only did this activity five days this week):

(_____ + _____ + _____ + _____ + _____ = _____) ÷ 5 = _____

Dinner:

(_____ + _____ + _____ + _____ + _____ + _____ + _____ = _____) ÷ 7 = _____

To bed:

(_____ + _____ + _____ + _____ + _____ + _____ + _____ = _____) ÷ 7 = _____

Exercise:

(_____ + _____ + _____ + _____ + _____ + _____ + _____ = _____) ÷ 7 = _____

CALEB'S SOCIAL RHYTHM METRIC (SRM) #2: SETTING TARGET TIMES

Activity	Target Time	Sunday Time	Monday Time	Tuesday Time	Wednesday Time	Thursday Time	Friday Time	Saturday Time
Out of bed	7:30 a.m.	11 a.m.	6:17 a.m.	6:10 a.m.	6:45 a.m.	6:05 a.m.	6:05 a.m.	10:15 a.m.
First contact with other person		Noon	7:30 a.m.	7:30 a.m.	7:30 a.m.	7:30 a.m.	7:30 a.m.	11 a.m.
Start work/school/volunteer/family care		——	8 a.m.	8 a.m.	8 a.m.	8 a.m.	8 a.m.	——
Dinner		7:15 p.m.	6:15 p.m.	6 p.m.	6:30 p.m.	6:10 p.m.	6:10 p.m.	7:00 p.m.
To bed		1:30 a.m.	9:30 p.m.	11:30 p.m.	9:30 p.m.	11 p.m.	1:30 a.m.	Midnight
Exercise		Noon	4:30 p.m.	4:30 p.m.	4:45 p.m.	4:15 p.m.	4:30 p.m.	11 a.m.
Rate MOOD each day from –5 to +5 –5 = very depressed +5 = very elated		1	–2	–1	–2	–1	2	–1
Rate ENERGY LEVEL each day –5 = very slowed, fatigued +5 = very energetic, active		2	–2	–2	–2	0	1	–1

Check your calculations for Caleb's average times against the answers below.

Out of bed: 7:30 a.m.

First contact with another person: 8:45 a.m.

Start work/school: 8 a.m. (he only did it five times this week, so divide by five)

Dinner: 6:30 p.m.

To bed: 11:30 p.m. (remember to convert to military time)

Exercise: 3 p.m. (remember to convert to military time)

EXERCISE 5.2 Calculate Your SRM Average Times

After calculating average SRM times for Caleb, calculate your own average SRM times using your completed SRMs for the past seven days. If you have information for more than three days but fewer than seven, add up the values for the days that you have available, and then divide by the number of times you did the activity. If you did the activity on three or fewer days, skip the calculation. Don't forget to convert to military time if the activities took place in both the a.m. and p.m.

Out of bed:

(_____ + _____ + _____ + _____+ _____ +_____ + _____

= _____) ÷ _____ = _____

First contact with another person:

(_____ + _____ + _____ + _____+ _____ +_____ + _____

= _____) ÷ _____ = _____

Start work/school/volunteer work:

(_____ + _____ + _____ + _____+ _____ +_____ + _____

= _____) ÷ _____ = _____

Dinner:

(_____ + _____ + _____ + _____ + _____ + _____ + _____

= _____) ÷ ____ = _____

To bed:

(_____ + _____ + _____ + _____ + _____ + _____ + _____

= _____) ÷ ____ = _____

Other:

(_____ + _____ + _____ + _____ + _____ + _____ + _____

= _____) ÷ ____ = _____

Other:

(_____ + _____ + _____ + _____ + _____ + _____ + _____

= _____) ÷ ____ = _____

SRM targets for the next week. In general, it's best to use the calculated SRM average, or circadian midpoint, as your SRM target time because this aligns best with your current body clock settings. If your circadian midpoint for dinner is 6:30 p.m., it's likely that you'll feel hungry at the time (caveat: this may not be the case if you have a lot of variability in your dinner time). Although you may want to change those settings (e.g., change your out-of-bed time from 9 a.m. to 7 a.m.), it's best to make these changes gradually, ideally in shifts of no more than thirty minutes per week. Avoiding abrupt shifts in timing of your SRMs will allow your body clock to gradually adjust to the new schedule. Starting from your existing routines rather than imposing a new or "perfect" schedule on yourself from the outset protects your body from experiencing a big change in your internal body clock. If you make too many abrupt changes, you'll create jet-lag-like experiences for yourself, which could further destabilize your mood. It's also psychologically easier to start with small changes because change is hard!

Adjusting target times for real life. There will be occasions when your circadian midpoint is not a feasible SRM target time because it would fall at an inopportune time for you, such as in the middle of classes or during work. If that is the case, you'll have to make a practical choice to set a target time that works with your schedule, recognizing that your body may feel "off" until it gets used to the new times. For instance, if your "start work" average time is not when you're expected to start work in real life, you'll have to adjust your target time to accommodate your work schedule.

When setting your SRM target times for each activity, keep the following principles in mind:

- Try for regularity before shifting the time of an activity. Your initial goal should be to reset your body clock by doing activities at the same time every day, including weekends. Once you're on track with activity regularity, you can begin to slowly change the target time if desired (there will be more information about shifting target times in chapter 6).

- Aim for your average time, or circadian midpoint, but if that is not possible, adjust as needed.

- Avoid changing your target time by more than thirty minutes per week. If you make abrupt changes, you'll confuse your body clock and may experience jet-lag-like symptoms.

In reviewing their SRM averages, Caleb noticed that some of their circadian midpoints were at awkward times. A 7:30 wake-up time wasn't feasible for them during the week because they must be at work by 7:30 a.m. It explained, however, why they were so tired when they woke up in the mornings (i.e., at 6:15 a.m., their body clock said it was time to sleep but the alarm clock said it was time to wake up). They realized they would need to keep 6:15 a.m. as their target time—which meant that they would eventually need to get up much earlier on the weekends to avoid inducing jet-lag-like confusion for their body clock come Monday morning. Times for starting work, dinner, and bedtime were okay, but their average exercise time, 3 p.m., was not possible during the week because of work. They decided they would set 4:30 p.m. as their target time for exercise—but that would mean exercising later in the day on the weekends. They felt like an 11:30 p.m. to-bed time was a late target time for them on weekdays, but they decided to leave it as their target bedtime for now to avoid making too many body clock shifts.

How do I decide which activity to focus on? Over time, your goal is to get to the point where you're doing most activities within forty-five minutes of your target time, as many days as possible but at least five or six days a week. To get started, record all your target times on your SRM so you know what you're working toward eventually. However, it's neither practical nor healthy to radically change your whole schedule all at once. *I recommend setting a goal for just one activity per week.* For example, you might start with your time out of bed—then, once it's stabilized, move to first contact with another person. Once that is going well, work on your start time for usual activity. You might reserve focusing on dinner time and bedtime until you have consistency in the other routines. You may also find that as some activities fall into place, others naturally follow.

Start with something that feels doable. Rather than focusing on the activity that is most irregular, start with one that you think you can be very consistent with over the week. Also, don't feel like this is a huge decision! Think about this as "I'll try it for a week and see how I feel." Approach target setting with a sense of curiosity rather than rigid expectations. No matter what happens, you'll learn about yourself, your routines, and your mood.

EXERCISE 5.3 Calculate Your SRM Target Times

Let's get started with target times! Use your calculated SRM averages (or best guesses for averages if the math business was too much), adjusted for the realities of your schedule, to identify all five of your SRM target times (seven, if you added two personal anchors). Try to select times that are as close to your circadian midpoint as possible. Think of these target times as benchmarks and aspirational goals that you'll work toward over the next few weeks. This week you should focus on *just one goal*. Which activity would you like to start with? In selecting your first goal, you might want to consider which feels manageable, which feels most important, or which you have had past successes with. You can also pick a random goal. Time out of bed is a good place to start if you don't feel strongly about another item. There is no wrong choice! In the spaces below, write down target times for each of the five SRM activities. Circle the one activity that you plan to focus on this week, with the goal of doing that activity within forty-five minutes of your target time on as many days as possible.

Out of bed: _____

First contact with another person: _____

Start work/school/volunteer work: _____

Dinner: _____

To bed: _____

Other: _____

Other: _____

Once you have established your SRM target times for the week, transfer them to your SRM form. These SRM target times will guide your SRM work for the next week.

Establishing "other" targets. On your SRM, there is space for two customized activities. This enables you to personalize your SRM to include activities that are important to you and part of your regular daily routines. You don't have to add anything to the "other" section, but you're welcome to do so. If you add something to the "other" row, be sure it's something that you do (almost) every day. You would calculate your target times for these activities just as you would for the five core SRM activities.

Meeting your targets. Now that you have set your SRM targets and selected a goal for the next week, you should start thinking about changes that you'll make to achieve regularity (within a forty-five-minute window) for your selected activity. How will you make the changes in your life so that you can meet your goal? How can you remember to stay on a new routine? Here are some strategies that will help you meet your goal:

- Check your SRM each morning when you wake up and each night before you go to bed. By glancing at your targets, you'll be reminded of your daily goals.

- Write your goal down somewhere and put it in a place where you'll see it, such as on a note card posted on the bathroom mirror or in your phone. Make sure you look at it to remind you of your goal.

- Set daily alarms on your phone to remind you when it's time for specific activities.

- Ask a friend or family member to remind you of your goal/target times.

- Remember that you're focusing on just a single activity this week. You can look at other activities and targets, but don't feel obligated to meet them.

Specific change strategies for each SRM activity. Once you have selected an activity that you wish to focus on, consider some of the specific recommendations (below) for each activity. You may wish to mark this section and return to it as you add SRM activities to your weekly goals. As a reminder, don't try to do all of this at once!

- *Out of bed.* From a circadian standpoint, this is the most important activity of the day. It anchors all the rest of your routines. If you aren't sure which activity to pick first, "out of bed" is always a good place to start. For many people, it's hard to stick to the same wake-up time on weekends. Yet, it really is important to get up at the same time on the weekends as you do on the weekdays to stabilize your body clock. If that isn't feasible, minimize the difference between your weekend and weekday wake-up times (e.g., a one-hour difference rather than a three-hour difference). Set lots of alarms (see chapter 8 for more tips on getting out of bed).

- *First contact with another person.* If you're having trouble connecting with someone each day at the same time, try reaching out to the people in your social network. Is there anyone who might be sympathetic to your "cause" of trying to add regular social interactions to your day? Who would you like to spend more time with? Who could you invite to meet you for coffee in the morning? A walk in the afternoon? A shared meal at dinner? Although social media may help you feel connected, face-to-face communication is important to our body clocks. Our bodies were "programmed" long before smartphones and computers were created, so it's unclear whether the hormones in our body respond to human contact via technology the same way it does when we're in a room with another human being. Try to find a regular time to be face-to-face with people.

- *Start an activity at the same time every day.* It's important to find something to do every day, but this can be especially challenging if you're not working or going to school. Although your long-term goal may be to return to school or work or to find a volunteer job, focus first on scheduling a "temporary" activity every day like meeting a friend, going for a walk, buying tickets for a movie in advance (so you're committed to going) or paying for a session with a trainer at the gym (again, so that you feel obligated to go). The internet can be a good source of ideas for activities. It's important to schedule activities on the weekends too, especially if you already have scheduled activities during the week but none on the weekends. Otherwise, your body clock slows down over the weekend, and you'll feel "off" by Monday morning.

- *Eat dinner at a regular time every day.* Dinner time helps to set our sleep time, organizing body clocks for nighttime. Dinners can be quick and easy. Don't worry about preparing a feast. It's fine to eat something small, light, and easy to prepare. Focus on eating something (anything!) at the same time every evening—including weekends. Plan to meet a friend for "a bite" or meal prep together. Setting an alarm on your phone to remind you to begin meal preparation might help you remember on Saturday and Sunday.

- *To bed.* Going to bed at a regular time every night helps to anchor your body clock. Some tips for going to bed at a regular time include developing a "wind-down" ritual, such as a warm bath, turning off computers, TVs, and bright lights at least an hour before bedtime, avoiding caffeine after noon, and making sure that your bedroom is dark, cool, and comfortable (more on this in chapter 8). Since time out of bed sets your sleep time, it's usually better and easier to work on regularizing your time out of bed before focusing on time to bed.

EXERCISE 5.4 Barriers and Solutions to Meeting SRM Targets

As with starting an exercise routine, stopping smoking, or losing weight, most of us struggle to change our behaviors, even when we think it could be healthy for us. It's common to put it off ("I'll start my diet next week"), feel overwhelmed ("there's no way I can get to the gym every day so why bother trying?"), or make excuses ("I don't really need to stop smoking—everyone around me smokes"). The same is true when we start making changes to our daily routines; procrastination and avoidance are common. Since it's normal to hesitate when starting to work on SRM targets, it can be helpful to do some anticipatory problem-solving before beginning. What are some barriers to change that you might encounter as you work toward your target times? How can you solve potential barriers to change?

Below is a list of common barriers to meeting SRM targets. Check all that apply to you. In the space provided, brainstorm ideas to overcoming the barrier. If you can't think of any solutions, don't worry about it; there are suggestions for managing barriers at the end of the exercise and additional suggestions in later chapters. If you would like to repeat this exercise, you can find a printable copy of it on the website for this book: http://www.newharbinger.com/51246.

☐ My target times are unrealistic: _____

_____

☐ I'm not in charge of preparing dinner so I have no control over my dinner time:

_____

_____

☐ I set my out-of-bed time one hour earlier than my circadian midpoint, and I never seem to make my target:

_____

_____

☐ I can't seem to stay within the recommended forty-five-minute window for my targets:

_____

_____

☐ I feel overwhelmed by all these targets: _____

_____

☐ I'm good; I don't have any trouble meeting my SRM targets.

Here are some tips to help you meet your target times. Check the ones that might be helpful for you.

☐ Use your social supports. It's always easier to meet goals when you have a buddy helping you. If your goal is to exercise daily at the same time, pair up with a friend who shares your goals. Meet up at the same time every day for walks or an exercise class. Or plan to meet a friend for dinner.

☐ Find an SRM coach. Behavior change is more effective when we hold ourselves accountable to another person.[85] Identify someone with whom you can share your goals and your progress each day. Your SRM coach can be a friend, relative, or a therapist.

☐ Eat a snack rather than dinner. If the idea of preparing dinner is overwhelming or if you rely on someone else for meals, have a small meal or a snack at the same time every day. You're sending an important signal to your intestinal body clocks even if you eat only a small amount of food.

☐ Break the goal into smaller pieces. If your ultimate goal is to set a wake-up time that is an hour earlier than your circadian midpoint, start by trying to get up thirty minutes earlier. If that is too hard, try for fifteen minutes earlier or five minutes earlier.

☐ Keep it simple. Try keeping your routines regular for just a few days rather than the whole week and see what you notice.

☐ Look at your mood and energy ratings to see if the changes you're making help your symptoms.

☐ Don't fixate on the forty-five-minute window. If sticking to the forty-five-minute window is too hard or your targets seem unrealistic, increase the window to sixty minutes or ninety minutes. Start with a goal that seems manageable. You can always shrink the window later, as you get more experience with this approach.

☐ Give yourself a break. If you're depressed, it's harder to work on tasks. Low energy and low motivation are symptoms of depression. It will take a bit longer to get where you want to go, but you'll get there.

☐ Reward yourself. If you can stick to your target time two days in a row, indulge in something pleasurable like watching a movie or taking a relaxing bath. If you manage to do five days in a row, go out for coffee with a friend or post your victory on social media.

List two things that you might try if you encounter barriers to reaching your SRM target.

1. I will _____

2. I will _____

Working on target times is marathon, not a sprint. Getting yourself on a regular schedule takes time. You should work on one target this week and then another target next week. Gradually, you'll bring your schedule into alignment with your targets. You can also adjust your targets over time. For instance, if you succeed in getting up most days at 10 a.m. but want to aim for an earlier time, you can gradually move your target time back by thirty minutes per week. As you continue to adjust your SRM targets over time, you don't have to go back through the process of calculating average times for the week; just gradually adjust your target times to fit your social rhythm goals. We'll discuss setting longer term social rhythm goals in the next chapter.

Summary. In this chapter, you learned to calculate circadian midpoints and set target times for your SRM. You now have tools to change some routines to increase social rhythm regularity. It's important to remember, however, that change takes time. You should not expect yourself to reach all your targets right away. Taking a stepwise approach to change (one activity at time) is more realistic and healthier for your circadian system. Once you've met one target, you can move on to the next.

In the next chapter, you'll learn how to set additional social rhythm goals. You'll start working on bigger picture social rhythm goals like finding a job with more regular hours or introducing regular exercise into your schedule. Setting these goals will help you take the next steps toward stabilizing your social rhythms, thereby improving your mood.

CHAPTER 6

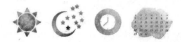

Setting Social Rhythm Goals

In this chapter, you'll build on earlier exercises from this book to discover common patterns of disruptions in social rhythms, learning how to detect them using your SRMs. You'll have opportunities to find these patterns in someone else's SRM (see "LaVonnie's SRM" below) and then you'll look for patterns in your own SRM. This will allow you to set some short-term and long-term social rhythm goals for yourself. Finding—and ultimately addressing—rhythm disruptions in your life will help you achieve overall routine stability and a more stable mood.

Social Rhythm Metric check-in. Before taking a deeper dive into your social rhythm patterns, take a minute to revisit your SRM from the past week. What do you notice about the connections between the regularity of your routines last week and your mood? Your energy levels? Have you been able to log your daily activities, mood, and energy? If not, what are some of the challenges you have faced? Can you think of any solutions to those challenges? (Hint: Look back at chapter 5 to find some suggestions for problem-solving barriers to SRM completion.)

What was it like to work on your first SRM goal? Did you achieve your goal or are you still working on it? If you didn't reach your goal, what are some strategies you might use this week to get closer to your goal? If you've achieved your first goal, what will you choose for your next goal?

Note that it may be helpful to build on prior successes. For instance, if you have successfully gotten up at the same time every day within a forty-five-minute window, you might want to work on backing up your wake-up time by thirty minutes. Or, perhaps you're ready to tackle making sure that you start an activity every day of the week at the same time, including weekends. Picking an

SRM goal for the week is a personal decision with no right or wrong choices. Write down your reflections on the past week's social rhythms and SRM goal for the upcoming week:

_____

_____

_____

_____

_____

_____

Common patterns of social rhythm disruption. With SRM goal-setting, we typically focus on one activity at time. To promote stable routines and stable moods, it's also important to look at broader patterns in your schedules. For instance, you may be the kind of person who has an overall regular schedule. In that case, you may use your SRM to tweak and maintain rhythm stability. Or, you may be the kind of person who is juggling lots of activities and whose schedule varies wildly from day to day and week to week. In that case, you may need to think about some of the big picture factors (e.g., two jobs, young children, limited social supports) that are contributing to your routine (in)stability. Just as no two people are the same, no one's social routines are identical. Here are some common patterns of social rhythm disruption to be on the lookout for if you have bipolar disorder:

- *Erratic routines.* No consistent routine day to day.

- *Shifted routines.* Tending toward getting up later and going to sleep later than others. You may go to sleep *later* at night than you "should" and then have trouble getting up in the mornings. Circadian experts call this pattern "phase-delayed" rhythms. They can also be shifted in the other direction (going to sleep very early and getting up very early—called "phase advanced"), but this is less common in bipolar disorder.

- *Inconsistent routines.* Keeping some rhythms consistent during the week, especially those with social expectancy (e.g., getting up for work, getting dinner on the table for your family), but struggling for consistency with other routines, especially those that lack strong social anchors (e.g., exercise, time to bed).

- *Social jet lag.* Social jet lag is a term used to describe the phenomenon of our bodies experiencing a misalignment between our natural circadian rhythms and our social obligations.[86] It occurs when we go to bed and wake up at different times on workdays versus days off or weekends. It can cause feelings of fatigue, irritability, and mood disturbances.

- *Gaps in the SRM.* Absence of regular daily activities and limited social contacts are common when you're struggling with depression. On the SRM, this is noticeable as "gaps" where you have nothing to record since you didn't do the activity.

We discuss below strategies for addressing each social rhythm pattern. Of course, some individuals with bipolar disorder have very regular routines. If you're very regular with your routines and if your mood and energy levels are stable, you're on the right track. SRT can help you preserve the regular routines that are working for you.

EXERCISE 6.1 Looking for Common Social Rhythm Patterns

This exercise will identify common patterns of social rhythm disruption in your life. First, you'll be asked to identify common patterns of rhythm disruption in an SRM example ("LaVonnie's SRM"). Then, you'll be asked to look at your own SRM to see what kinds of patterns you notice.

LaVonnie is an eighteen-year-old college student, identifies as female, uses she/her pronouns, and has bipolar II disorder. LaVonnie goes to classes during the week and likes to socialize with friends on weekends. Her classes start at 8:30 a.m. on Mondays, Wednesdays, and Fridays and at 10:30 a.m. on Tuesdays. She doesn't have class on Thursdays or the weekend. She takes medications for bipolar disorder at night and tracks this on her SRM to help her remember. She also tracks the time that she starts doing her homework each day.

LAVONNIE'S SOCIAL RHYTHM METRIC (SRM)

Activity	Target Time	Sunday Time	Monday Time	Tuesday Time	Wednesday Time	Thursday Time	Friday Time	Saturday Time
Out of bed		Noon	8 a.m.	10 a.m.	8 a.m.	10:30 a.m.	8 a.m.	11 a.m.
First contact with other person		Noon	8:30 a.m.	10:30 a.m.	8:30 a.m.	11 a.m.	8:30 a.m.	11 a.m.
Start work/school/ volunteer/family care		----	8:30 a.m.	10:30 a.m.	8:30 a.m.	----	8:30 a.m.	----
Dinner		----	7 p.m.	6 p.m.	6:30 p.m.	8 p.m.	8 p.m.	7 p.m.
To bed		1:30 a.m.	11:30 p.m.	11:30 p.m.	9:30 p.m.	11 p.m.	3 a.m.	1:30 a.m.
Homework		8 p.m.	2:30 p.m.	2:30 pm	4 p.m.	11:30 a.m.	----	----
Take medications		Midnight	11 p.m.	11 p.m.	----	10:30 p.m.	2:45 a.m.	1:30 a.m.
Rate MOOD each day from −5 to +5 −5 = very depressed +5 = very elated		−1	−2	−2	0	−1	2	−1
Rate ENERGY LEVEL each day −5 = very slowed, fatigued +5 = very energetic, active		−2	−2	0	−2	−1	−1	−1

In LaVonnie's SRM, which of the following common social rhythm disruption patterns do you notice? Check all that apply. In the space next to the checked item, write down your observations. See the example below to help you get started:

☑ Erratic routines *There is no consistent activity, except maybe dinner, but even that has a two-hour range, which is a lot of variability.*

☐ Shifted routines _____

_____

☐ Inconsistent routines _____

_____

☐ Social jet lag _____

_____

☐ Gaps in the SRM _____

_____

As a college student, LaVonnie has a lot of irregularity in her routines. LaVonnie gets up at different times each day, depending on when she has classes. An inconsistent wake-up time sets the stage for *erratic routines*. It's hard for her to maintain consistency with any of her routines, including taking her medication at a regular time (notice that she even missed her medications on Wednesday night). She seems to gravitate toward *phase-delayed routines*, getting up later when left to her own schedule (e.g., when she doesn't have an early class) and staying up late most evenings. There is a mismatch between her weekend schedule and weekday schedule, especially around her sleep and wake times. This suggests that LaVonnie experiences *social jet lag*. Finally, there are some *gaps* in her SRM, especially on the days when she doesn't have classes. Not surprisingly, her mood and energy levels are affected by these erratic routines.

Which of the following common rhythm disruptions do you experience? Check all that apply. Add comments describing what you notice in your life.

☐ Erratic routines _____

_____

☐ Shifted routines _____

_____

☐ Inconsistent routines _____

_____

☐ Social jet lag _____

_____

☐ Gaps in my SRM _____

_____

Write down observations about your overall SRM patterns, including the relationships among your SRM patterns, mood, and energy ratings:

_____

_____

_____

_____

_____

Tips for managing irregular SRM patterns. If you have noticed irregular patterns in your daily life, you can start setting goals to address these issues. This may be in addition to or instead of your weekly SRM goal. Irregular patterns in your life may require rethinking multiple aspects of your weekly routines or making bigger picture changes in your life.

Below are some tips for managing common patterns of social rhythm disruption:

- *Erratic routines.* It may be important to think about some of the "bigger picture" factors, such as jobs, family, and social supports, that contribute to your difficulty establishing regular routines. Exercises 6.2 and 6.3 will help you with this. You may need to be gentle with yourself about your routines until you're able to address some of the environmental factors that make it hard to stay regular. In the meantime, it may be helpful to focus on one "doable" item on the SRM (e.g., first contact with another person or exercise) to introduce at least some regularity into your life.

- *Shifted routines.* In chapter 1, we discussed chronotype. Tending toward late nights and late mornings describes the "night owl" chronotype, as is common for those with bipolar disorder. In general, we try not to fight biology. So, if you have an owl-ish chronotype, it's best to establish a *regular but later* schedule. For instance, working a job that goes from noon to 8 p.m. may feel more natural than fighting your natural rhythms to work a 9–5 job. If, however, you absolutely must get up and get going earlier than you would like (e.g., for childcare or a specific job), you should focus on your time out of bed. This routine has the strongest pull on our circadian rhythms, so being especially conscientious about this social rhythm will help you stay on track, despite your chronotype. Biology will always pull you toward later routines, however, so you'll have to be extra vigilant with your time out of bed (including on weekends!) if you wish to remain on an earlier schedule.

- *Inconsistent routines.* If some of your routines are more consistent than others, it may be paradoxically better to focus first on those that are more regular. For instance, if you're pretty good about a regular dinnertime but are inconsistent with bedtime, it may be best to focus on dinnertime for a few weeks to make sure it's "rock solid" before tackling bedtime. The rationale for this is that circadian rhythms are interconnected. Eating dinner at a consistent time sends a signal to your brain that night-time will be starting soon. So, making sure that your dinnertime is consistent can help provide needed information to your brain to help regularize bedtime. You can find additional strategies for stabilizing bedtime (once dinnertime is going well!) in chapter 8.

- *Social jet lag.* To combat social jet lag, it's essential to prioritize a consistent sleep schedule and limit disruptions to other routines, especially on the weekends. Finding an SRM buddy to help you stick to your schedule on weekends can help fight off feelings of isolation if your schedule differs from those around you on Saturdays and Sundays.

- *Gaps in my SRM.* Having blank spots in your weekly SRM is not uncommon. Although the occasional skipped or absent item is not usually a problem for achieving social rhythm (and therefore mood) stability, having a pattern of lots of missed or absent items can be problematic. This "swiss cheese" SRM pattern suggests that you may not have enough commitments or connections to anchor your life. First, identify which SRM item has the most blanks and brainstorm ways to plug the gaps. For instance, if you have many days without contacting another person, make a list of people in your life who may be willing to meet for a meal, coffee, or walk. If you can't identify anyone in your social networks who could help, consider plan B options like interacting with a barista at a local coffee shop or texting a friend. Once you have reduced gaps on one SRM item, move on to the next. But, again, do this in a stepwise fashion, perhaps one goal per week.

EXERCISE 6.2 Circumstances That Help or Hurt Routines

In addition to the five items tracked on the SRM, broader life circumstances impact your overall social rhythm regularity. Therefore, it's important to think about and develop strategies to address conditions in your life that contribute to rhythm regularity (or irregularity). For instance, if you work different shifts every day, it will be very hard to establish regular routines without rethinking your job situation. If you don't have a job and don't go to school, it's hard to establish a regular routine unless you add a daily commitment such as volunteering or a gym class. The following exercise (6.3) will encourage you to think about life factors that either help or hurt your rhythm regularity. This exercise will help you consider strategies that may help you achieve regular daily routines in the face rhythm-disturbing life circumstances.

Below are common social factors that affect regularity of routines and therefore moods. In the space below, reflect on how these issues either promote regularity (help) or cause rhythm disruption (hurt) in your life. The first item is filled out to give you an example. You can also write "N/A" if the item is not applicable to you. There are spaces for you to add additional activities. Note that the focus for this exercise is *the impact of the circumstances on your routines*, not whether you overall like it. For instance, you may love your nursing job but also recognize that its irregular shifts and forced overtime hurt your routines. Or you may be thrilled to have four small children, but also recognize that caring for them makes it very hard for you to do anything at the same time every day.

Activity	Helps Routines	Hurts Routines
Pet	I get up every morning at 7 a.m. to walk my dog–no matter the weather. I also walk him at 5 p.m. before dinner.	My dog takes up a lot of space in my bed at night. It makes it hard for me to sleep so I am very tired.
Job		
School		
Children		

Activity	Helps Routines	Hurts Routines
Parents		
Partner		
Friend(s)		
Physical health		
Living situation		
Finances		

EXERCISE 6.3 Short-Term and Long-Term Goals

Once you've identified circumstances in your life that disrupt routines, you can develop goals for these circumstances that may help you achieve more regularity in your life. Of course, some circumstances may not be immediately changeable (e.g., small children will grow up over the next decade, but there is no possibility of making them grow up faster). But others may be ripe for change (e.g., starting an exercise routine or negotiating at work for more regular shifts). Think about your priorities and then check the boxes listing goals that may be relevant to you. Indicate whether you would like to achieve the goal in the short term (one to three weeks) or long term (three months to one year). For example, you may decide that "go to bed at the same time every night" is a good short-term goal for you, whereas "get a new job" is relevant but should be considered a long-term goal. You can also check "N/A" if a goal is not applicable to you. There is space to add personal goals at the end.

Goal	Short-Term	Long-Term	Does not apply
Get a pet to help me get up on time			
Make some new friends so I have someone to see every day			
Join a gym/exercise regularly			
Get a volunteer job so I have somewhere I need to be every day			
Get a new job with regular hours			
Go to bed at the same time every night			
Get more involved with religious activities so I have more activities in my life			
Get some roommates so that I have more social contacts			
Go back to school so that I have somewhere I need to be			
Ask my romantic partner to help me stick to a schedule			
Learn how to cook so I can make dinner for myself at the same time every night			
Ask my parents to help me stay on a regular schedule			
Find more home care for my elderly parents so I don't have to spend so many nights away from home to help them			

EXERCISE 6.4 Achieving a Short-Term Goal

Pick one or two short-term goals from exercise 6.3 that you would like to work on and note them here:

_____

_____

Once you have identified your goal(s), think about steps you can take to meet your goal(s). As with SRM targets, you should start with small steps. For instance, if your goal is to get more involved with your church, synagogue, or mosque so that you have more scheduled activities and social contacts, start with something easy, such as looking at the website to learn more about their offerings (goal #1). Then, maybe ask a friend to go with you to a single worship-related activity (goal #2). If that goes well, consider going twice during the following week (goal #3). Eventually you might wish to build up to committing to a recurring class (religious text study class, social events) or even volunteering. Here are some tips that you can use to help achieve your goal:

- Break the goal into small pieces. If your goal is to get a pet, start by visiting an animal shelter or volunteering to care for a friend or neighbor's pet for a short period as a first goal, building up to your main goal.

- Use your social supports. It's always easier to meet goals when you have a buddy helping you. If your goal is to exercise regularly, pair up with a friend who shares your goal. Meet up for walks or take an exercise class together.

- Reward progress. When you make progress, give yourself a small "gift." If your goal is to get a volunteer job and you successfully pushed yourself to make several "dreaded" calls to ask about opportunities, reward yourself with a pleasurable activity like a comforting bath, an interesting podcast, or an enjoyable walk.

What are strategies you can use to meet your short-term goal? List what you plan to do first, second, and third to meet your goal. Remember to work on your goal in a stepwise fashion!

1. _____

2. _____

3. _____

EXERCISE 6.5 Deciding on a Long-Term Goal

If it's difficult for you to make changes, it might be enough to focus just on a short-term goal. If you're eager to keep going, however, this exercise will guide you toward a long-term goal. It's perfectly fine to skip this exercise if you feel like you already have enough on your plate.

Before embarking on a big life change, it's important to ask yourself questions about the proposed change to ensure that this is something that you really want to pursue. You should ponder how important it is to you, consider the pros and cons of enacting the change, and think about how it will affect your routines. The following prompts will help you consider whether this is a goal you wish to pursue.

What is a long-term goal that you would like to work on?

_____

How will this goal help you achieve better regularity of routines? Better moods?

_____

_____

How *important* is it to you to make this change? _____

How *likely* is it that you'll be able to make this change? _____

What are the pros of making the change? _____

_____

What are the cons of making the change? _____

_____

What discomforts are you willing to tolerate to enact the change?

_____

_____

Do you want to commit to making this change? If so, why now?

_____

_____

_____

If, after considering the questions above, you've decided it's worthwhile to work on this long-term goal and you're ready to commit to it, exercise 6.6 will help you successfully reach your goal. If, however, after answering these questions, you decide that this is not the right goal for you, then pause. You can go back to your lists in exercises 6.2 and 6.3 to see if there is another option. Go through this exercise again to consider carefully this second option. If the second option works for you, great! Proceed to exercise 6.6. If, however, you're still not sure you want to pursue a long-term goal right now, set exercise 6.6 aside until you feel ready to come back to it. You'll have chances to work on long-term goals in the future.

EXERCISE 6.6 Working on a Long-Term Goal

Even more so than with short-term goals, you should break down long-term goals into small pieces. Below, you'll be asked to break your long-term goal into a series of smaller steps and identify a time frame for achieving each step. It's helpful to be very specific about your goals and indicate a reasonable time frame for completing the activity. For instance, instead of saying you'll "call some people," write down that you'll "call two people from my old job by next Thursday." Here is an example of the kind of steps you might take to meet the goal of finding a new job with a better or more regular schedule:

1. Look at job postings in my field online (November 1)

2. Reach out by email to one person at the company that I'm interested in to make sure that hours are as regular as advertised (November 7)

3. Update my resume (November 15)

4. Send in one job application (December 1)

5. Send in five more job applications (December 31)

6. Follow up with two social contacts by email for additional advice on job hunting if not yet successful (January 15)

Outline steps that you'll take to reach a long-term goal below. Remember to include dates by which you hope to reach each goal.

This is my goal: _____

Here are the steps (in order) that I'll take, with dates:

1. _____

2. _____

3. _____

4. _____

5. _____

Despite best intentions, sometimes we're unable to meet goals we set for ourselves. Completing tasks can be especially challenging when you don't feel well. Rather than feeling discouraged, you might want to return to exercise 6.5 to consider whether this goal remains important to you at this time. If not, feel free to set it aside. If you still want to move ahead but find you're struggling to meet your goal, try revisiting the tips outlined in exercise 6.4, including asking for help from your social supports and rewarding yourself for small increments in progress. Especially if you're feeling depressed, set very small goals and give yourself a big pat on the back each time you accomplish a goal, no matter how small. Check your SRMs to see if your mood changes (hopefully for the better) as you make even small changes to work toward your social rhythm regularity goals.

Summary. In this chapter, we moved from micro (e.g., time out of bed) to macro (e.g., jobs and family) social rhythms. You learned how to identify patterns of irregularity in your SRM and considered how current life circumstances impact your daily routines. In addition to setting social rhythm goals using the SRM, you identified both short- and long-term social rhythm goals. Throughout, we underscored the importance of sequencing your goals so that you don't take on too much at once. As a reminder, you should go on this journey at your own pace, adding goals only when you feel ready.

The next two chapters will focus on sleep. In chapter 7, you'll learn how your body regulates sleep. In chapter 8, you'll develop strategies to improve your sleep.

CHAPTER 7

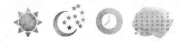

Sleep: What You Need to Know

This chapter and the one that follows focus on sleep. When you have bipolar disorder, your sleep-wake cycle is central to wellness. Sleep, by definition, is a problem during mood episodes (usually too much during depressive episodes and too little during mania). Sleep disruptions are themselves risk factors for new mood episodes. Even when feeling well, many people with bipolar disorder have trouble with sleep. By contrast, consistent, high-quality sleep is associated with mood stability. Chapter 7 provides you with information about how sleep works in your brain and body. Chapter 8 focuses on specific changes you can make to improve your sleep.

Before getting started with sleep, however, let's revisit your social rhythm stability so far. Because SRT skills build on each other, it's helpful to review changes that you have already made before adding a focus on sleep. Hopefully, you'll be pleasantly surprised to see how far you have come.

EXERCISE 7.1 Assessing Progress

To assess your SRT progress, rate the extent to which you agree with the following statements. You can find a printable copy of this exercise on the website for this book at http://www.newharbinger.com/51246 to redo this exercise over time.

I have increased the regularity of my daily routines.

Strongly Agree_____   Agree_____   Undecided_____   Disagree_____   Strongly Disagree_____

I can identify the symptoms of bipolar disorder.

Strongly Agree_____   Agree_____   Undecided_____   Disagree_____   Strongly Disagree_____

I know how to evaluate my SRMs.

Strongly Agree_____   Agree_____   Undecided_____   Disagree_____   Strongly Disagree_____

I feel comfortable rating my mood on a –5 to +5 scale.

Strongly Agree_____   Agree_____   Undecided_____   Disagree_____   Strongly Disagree_____

I have successfully completed at least one social rhythm goal.

Strongly Agree_____   Agree_____   Undecided_____   Disagree_____   Strongly Disagree_____

I recognize the link between daily rhythms and moods in my own life.

Strongly Agree_____   Agree_____   Undecided_____   Disagree_____   Strongly Disagree_____

I can identify *stabilizing* social rhythm anchors in my life.

Strongly Agree_____   Agree_____   Undecided_____   Disagree_____   Strongly Disagree_____

I can recognize and anticipate *disrupting* social rhythm factors in my life.

Strongly Agree_____   Agree_____   Undecided_____   Disagree_____   Strongly Disagree_____

I can get my life back on track after a social rhythm disruption.

Strongly Agree_____   Agree_____   Undecided_____   Disagree_____   Strongly Disagree_____

I have very regular daily routines.

Strongly Agree_____   Agree_____   Undecided_____   Disagree_____   Strongly Disagree_____

Consider your responses to the questions above. For which items did you choose "strongly agree" or "agree"? Note these items below:

_____

These are probably areas where you have made a lot of progress in SRT. Nice work!

For which items did you choose "undecided" or "disagree" or "strongly disagree"? Note these items below:

_____

These are areas that you're probably still working on. It's expected that you will not have mastered all components of SRT; it takes time! Here are some tips to help you continue to make progress in SRT, especially in the areas that continue to be challenging:

- Revisit information contained in earlier chapters. For instance, if you're still unsure about the symptoms of bipolar disorder, try rereading chapter 2. To remind yourself about the links between body clocks and moods, revisit chapter 1.

- Keep reading this book. Future chapters provide more information about social rhythms and additional strategies to help you manage them effectively. As you continue reading this book, you'll improve your mastery of SRT.

- Keep paying attention to links among body clocks, daily rhythms, and moods. Look for examples in your daily life. For instance, when you got stuck at work late this week, what happened to your dinner time? Your bedtime? Your mood? What happened when you successfully stayed on a regular routine?

- Continue to complete your SRM. Look for patterns in your SRM, especially links between regularity and mood. Pay attention to what changes on your SRM as you reach your social rhythm goals.

Remember that change is hard, and finding mood stability is a journey. If you continue to work on these challenges, you'll continue to make progress in SRT!

What is the relationship between sleep and bipolar disorders? If you have bipolar disorder, you have probably experienced sleep disturbances, including difficulty falling asleep, waking up during the night, early-morning awakening, and oversleeping. Indeed, sleep disruptions are among the most common symptoms of bipolar mood episodes.[87] People with bipolar disorder who have sleep disturbances are more likely to experience mood episodes and have longer periods of illness than those who do not have sleep problems.[88] Thus, the relationship between sleep and bipolar disorder is bidirectional, with poor sleep putting you at risk for new mood episodes and mood episodes putting you at risk for poor sleep.

Why do humans sleep? We spend one third of our lives asleep, and yet the fundamental purpose of sleep remains unclear. Some scientists think sleep helps promote growth of nerve cell communication (synapses), and others think it helps to prune these connections.[89] Newer research suggests that sleep helps the brain to clean itself, removing toxins and metabolic waste.[90] Regardless of its primary biologic functions, good-quality sleep is associated with wellness, whereas disturbances in sleep are associated with negative behavioral and physical health effects.[91] Good-quality sleep for most adults means seven to nine hours of relatively undisturbed sleep,[92] other than brief awakenings that last less than thirty minutes. Young children and adolescents need more sleep than midlife adults;[93] older adults need less.[94]

Despite its centrality to human functioning, sleep problems are common, including trouble falling asleep, trouble staying asleep, waking up too early in the morning, and sleeping too much. When your sleep is off, you feel irritable, lethargic, and foggy; your concentration is worse, your motivation is lower, and you have slower physical reaction times.[95] Poor sleep (both too little and too much) predisposes you to mood episodes, cardiovascular disease, diabetes, obesity, and even some cancers.[96] We need good-quality sleep to remain healthy.

EXERCISE 7.2 Assessing Sleep

Below is a list of common sleep problems. Check the kinds of sleep problem that pertain to you (check all that apply). In the space provided, make a note about whether you experienced these problems when depressed, (hypo) manic, or in a stable mood. You may have these sleep problems in more than one mood state.

☐ Trouble falling asleep   _____

☐ Trouble staying asleep   _____

☐ Multiple awakenings of at least thirty   _____
   minutes during the night

☐ Waking up very early, at least an hour   _____
   before you would have to get up

☐ Not enough sleep   _____

☐ Too much sleep   _____

☐ Trouble getting out of bed in the morning   _____

If you checked one or more sleep problems (many people with bipolar disorder check all of them), continue reading. You'll learn more about the relationship between sleep problems and bipolar disorder in the remainder of this chapter. In the following chapter, you'll learn strategies to address these issues.

What are the relationships among sleep, circadian rhythms, and bipolar disorder?

Melatonin, a hormone secreted by the pineal gland in your brain, and cortisol, a stress hormone produced by the adrenal glands in response to signals from the brain, play crucial roles in regulating sleep.[97] As daylight decreases and darkness sets in, signals are sent from the back of the eye to the master circadian clock of the brain, also known as the suprachiasmatic nucleus (SCN).[98] Genes in the SCN are turned on, expressing proteins that send messages to the nearby pineal gland to start producing melatonin.[99] Known as the "darkness hormone," melatonin levels increase throughout the night, peaking in the early morning hours. In parallel, levels of cortisol, also known as an "alerting hormone," fall at night and rise again in the morning.[100] Rising melatonin and dropping cortisol levels at night facilitate sleep by making us feel drowsy and less alert. They also help to regulate the timing and duration of sleep by promoting deeper, more restful sleep.[101]

Individuals with bipolar disorder have abnormalities in the circadian system during both well and ill periods.[102] Disruptions to circadian rhythms, including disturbances in melatonin and cortisol production, may contribute to the development and severity of bipolar disorder symptoms.[103] Although the precise mechanism by which bipolar disorder causes alterations in melatonin and cortisol secretion is unknown, it seems likely that sleep changes in bipolar disorder are at least partially related to disturbances in the normal patterns of these hormones.

What is sleep drive? Sleep drive or sleep pressure are ways to describe hormones and proteins that build up in your blood stream over the course of the day to make you feel sleepy.[104] Sleepiness occurs when enough factors related to sleep drive have accumulated in your body, including a protein called adenosine.[105] If levels of these factors are too low, you'll have trouble falling asleep. For most people, it takes fourteen to sixteen hours for enough sleep drive to accumulate to be able to fall asleep. That means that if you get up at 10 a.m., you probably won't feel sleepy until midnight, at the earliest. Sleeping during the middle of the day (i.e., naps) depletes your sleep drive, making it harder to fall asleep at night. By contrast, after maintaining alertness for sixteen hours, most of us start nodding off and find sleep hard to resist.

With rising and falling levels of sleep-promoting factors like melatonin and adenosine, our sleep drive helps keep us stable by keeping our sleep schedules regular. Once we fall asleep, sleep drive remains high for the first half of the night, but then starts to decrease. By morning, sleep drive levels are low. This explains, in part, why we don't go right back to sleep after a good night of sleep and how we're able to fall asleep at night, after being alert during the day. But sleep drive is only part of the biologic puzzle that regulates sleep.

How do circadian rhythms affect sleep? In addition to sleep drive, circadian rhythms play an important role in regulating sleep. Sleep researchers refer to this as a "two-process model of sleep,"[106] meaning that circadian-controlled factors such as timing of cortisol secretion work together with sleep drive to ensure optimal sleep. In an ideal world, sleep drive and circadian rhythms align to help you fall asleep. For instance, at 11 p.m., your body has built up enough sleep drive after sixteen hours of wakefulness to make you feel sleepy. At 11 p.m., your body clock supports sleep by secreting melatonin and shutting down other circadian functions that may interfere with sleep (e.g., elimination, hunger, focus/concentration). The opposite happens around 7 a.m., when sleep drive is depleted, melatonin is suppressed, and daytime circadian functions (such as cortisol) come back to life. You wake up refreshed, thanks to low levels of melatonin and sleep drive and higher levels of alerting factors.

What happens when sleep drive and circadian rhythms are misaligned? Sleep becomes disrupted when signals from your body clock and sleep drive are out of sync. Here are some examples:

- It's nighttime, and your body clock says, "Sleep!" Melatonin levels rise and non-sleep-related circadian functions slow. But, because you have only been awake for a few hours after a long nap or sleeping late in the morning, your sleep drive is low. Even though your body clock "knows" it's time to sleep, you toss and turn because you aren't yet tired enough to fall asleep. You feel both tired and not tired at the same time.

- It's morning, and your body clock says, "Wake up!" It's sunny outside, so your eyes tell your brain to tell your pineal gland to stop producing melatonin. You notice that you're hungry, and you feel the urge to go to the bathroom. However, you had a sleepless night (because of jet lag or shift work or a crying baby) and have been awake for many hours, increasing sleep pressure. So, you feel sleepy but also cannot fall back asleep because you're alert. You're both awake and not awake.

When your brain gets mixed messages from your circadian system and your sleep drive, sleep is usually disrupted or poor quality. Even though you're exhausted, you cannot fall asleep. Sometimes one process overrides the other—for example, finding yourself falling asleep in the middle of the day after an all-night trip to the emergency room—but until the two processes align, good sleep will remain elusive.

Bipolar disorder and sleep. As mentioned earlier, sleep and bipolar disorder are inextricably linked. During bipolar depressive episodes, energy and motivation are low. Typically, people oversleep when depressed. But, as a result, sleep drive remains low, even as night approaches. So, although you feel tired and the clock says 2 a.m., you toss and turn in your bed because sleep drive is low. Also, having bipolar disorder may throw off your body clock. This may result in a situation where you have built up plenty of sleep drive but your circadian system "tells" you that it's not yet time to sleep. Again, this can lead to trouble falling asleep and staying asleep. When manic, your brain remains "on" all night, making it hard to sleep at all. Thus, sleep problems are both caused by and characteristic of bipolar disorder.

All these experiences can create negative feedback loops such that trouble falling asleep and staying asleep will lead to a poor night's sleep, which will lead to naps and other behaviors that may disrupt sleep drive the next day. It can feel almost impossible to get out of these cycles, especially when your mood is poor and your energy is low. If you experience this feedback loop in your life, suggestions provided in the next chapter will help, so keep reading!

EXERCISE 7.3 How Can Sleep Go Wrong?

When you have bipolar disorder, there are many ways that sleep can go wrong, often the result of misalignment between circadian drive and sleep drive. Below are examples of common sleep problems in bipolar disorder. Check the scenarios that apply to you, either currently or in the past. Strategies provided in chapter 8 will help you find ways to address these concerns.

- ☐ *Going to bed too early.* You're depressed and exhausted. You crawl into bed at 10 p.m., having gotten up at noon. When you try to go to sleep at 10 p.m., however, you haven't given your body enough time to build up sufficient sleep drive. Although your energy level is low and your body clock tells you it's time to sleep, you're still wide awake as night falls. You probably won't fall asleep until fourteen hours after your wake time, or 2 a.m., because your circadian rhythms and sleep drive are misaligned.

☐ *Confused body clock.* Because you have a sensitive body clock, your body clock has trouble resetting itself after a change in environmental clocks (e.g., moving to daylight savings time or jet lag). Your body clock may "think" it's only 9 p.m., even though the external clock reads 1 a.m., making it hard to fall asleep or stay asleep. A mismatch between your body clock and the external clocks is common when you have bipolar disorder, and contributes to difficulty with sleep.

☐ *Taking long daytime naps.* If you have bipolar disorder, you may have the urge to take a long nap during the day because you're feeling depressed or because you had bad-quality sleep the night prior. However, taking naps during the day can interfere with the buildup of sleep drive, therefore making it hard to fall or stay asleep when circadian nighttime arrives.

☐ *Getting up at different times each morning.* In addition to input from light, the main circadian pacemaker in the SCN relies on feedback from circadian inputs throughout your body to determine when it's time to sleep. If you get up at different times each day, your body clock becomes confused about "when" it is, diminishing the intensity or amplitude of circadian signaling in your brain. With lower levels of circadian rhythmicity, you may have trouble falling or staying asleep. This problem is not specific to bipolar disorder, but it is harder to manage when you have a sensitive circadian pacemaker.

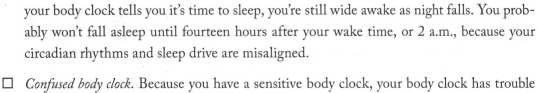

The first step to addressing sleep problems is to identify and understand them. By checking some (or all) of the scenarios above, you have started to recognize your sleep issues. The next chapter will help you solve them.

Does behavior affect sleep? In addition to misalignment of sleep drive and circadian rhythms, behavior also affects quality of sleep. Below are examples of common actions or activities that impact sleep:

• Drinking alcohol may make you feel relaxed or sleepy, but it ultimately disrupts the quality of sleep by changing sleep architecture, including lowering levels of restorative slow-wave sleep and increasing less restorative rapid eye movement sleep.[107] It's also a diuretic, which means that you'll wake up during the night to use the bathroom. Drinking relaxes the muscles in your body, including those in your throat and nose, which will make it more likely that you'll snore and sleep fitfully.

- Cannabis products are promoted as sleep aids, but evidence supporting their use for this purpose is limited. Cannabinoids affect the SCN, altering circadian rhythms in mice. Sleep difficulties are commonly identified as a byproduct of cannabis withdrawal, suggesting that regular use of these products worsens sleep.[108]

- The temperature of your bedroom at night affects sleep. Bedrooms that are too warm decrease slow-wave (restorative) sleep and promote wakefulness.[109] An ideal temperature for sleep is 65 degrees Fahrenheit.

- Exercise can both help and hurt sleep. Exercise during the day helps you sleep better,[110] but exercising too close to bedtime may interfere with sleep.

- Light at night worsens sleep. All screens (telephones, tablets, computers, televisions) emit blue spectrum light, a wavelength that our brains associate with daytime. Blue light suppresses melatonin secretion and promotes wakefulness. Therefore, if you look at screens too close to bedtime, you may be making your sleep worse. Conversely, evidence suggests that blocking blue light at night improves sleep,[111] including for those with bipolar disorder.[112]

EXERCISE 7.4 Helps or Hurts Sleep

Below is a list of activities that affect sleep for many people. Which activities or behaviors help you sleep better? Which hurt your sleep? For each activity or behavior, check whether it helps or hurts your sleep. You can check both boxes; you can also check that the activity does not apply to you. Add a comment about how the activity affects you (see example below). Write in any other sleep-related activities that you can think of at the bottom. Identifying activities or behaviors that help or hurt your sleep will help you start thinking about strategies you may want to reinforce or change to improve your sleep.

Activity/ Behavior	Helps My Sleep	Hurts My Sleep	Does Not Apply
Pets	Snuggling with my cat helps me fall asleep	My cat wakes me up at 4 a.m. to feed her	
Alcohol			

Activity/ Behavior	Helps My Sleep	Hurts My Sleep	Does Not Apply
Cannabis			
Nicotine			
Caffeine			
Exercise			
Temperature in bedroom			
Bedtime wind-down routine			
Time out of bed in morning			
Screen time at night			
Social media			
Spiritual practice/ meditation			
Reading			
Sex			

Activity/ Behavior	Helps My Sleep	Hurts My Sleep	Does Not Apply
Listening to music			
Journaling			
Pets			
Children			
Sleeping partner			

Summary. We started this chapter by assessing your progress in SRT. You identified areas that are going well for you and others that you would like to continue working on. You identified your personal challenges with sleep, including situations where sleep drive and circadian rhythms are misaligned.

The next chapter will continue to focus on sleep. Having learned about processes that control sleep and the unique barriers that make sleep difficult for you, you'll develop strategies to effectively improve your sleep. Improved sleep will contribute to improved health.

CHAPTER 8

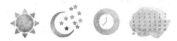

Improving Sleep with Social Rhythm Therapy

This chapter will give you tools to take control of your sleep. Following these strategies will help you maintain a more consistent sleep schedule and thereby stabilize your mood. But, as always, let's first check in on your social rhythm goals. To repeat this exercise, visit http://www.newharbinger. com/51246 for a printable copy.

Have you pursued your SRM and social rhythms goals this week? Did you achieve an SRM goal? A short-term goal? A long-term goal? Note below what you have accomplished so far.

_____

_____

Have you noticed connections between regularity of your SRM routines and your mood? As you've met your goals and moved toward more stable routines, have your mood and energy ratings changed? What are you noticing about the relationship between your mood and your SRMs? Make a few notes below.

_____

_____

What barriers have you encountered as you pursue your social rhythm goals? What are some strategies you might try in the upcoming days to address those barriers? (Hints: Break the goal into smaller pieces; reward yourself for taking steps toward regularity; be gentle with yourself if you're not yet ready to move forward.)

_____

_____

_____

_____

_____

_____

Are you ready to set a new goal? Perhaps pick a sleep-related goal since this chapter will help you find strategies to meet this goal. Write your new goal(s) here:

_____

_____

As we turn our attention to sleep, remember to continue to complete your SRM daily and work on your social rhythm goals.

EXERCISE 8.2 Sleep Hygiene

General sleep habits, also known as sleep hygiene, are daily routines that promote consistent, high-quality sleep. Although one size doesn't fit all when it comes to managing sleep problems and bipolar disorder, following well-established principles of sleep hygiene will help address many of the most common sleep issues associated with bipolar disorder. Below are tips for better sleep. Put a check mark (✓) next to the ones that you're already doing regularly. Put a plus (+) mark next to ones that you would like to implement to improve your sleep. Put an X next to those that don't apply or don't appeal to you.

✓, +, or X	Sleep Tip
	Make sure your bedroom is dark, quiet, and comfortable.
	Keep your room at a moderate temperature, around 65 degrees Fahrenheit.
	Eat regular meals, and do not go to sleep hungry.
	Avoid greasy foods at night.
	Only use the bedroom for sleep and sex.
	Don't take your problems to bed. Keep a journal nearby to write down "worry thoughts" before going to sleep.
	Develop a soothing bedtime routine like a warm bath, quiet music, or caffeine-free tea.
	Don't drink a lot of liquids in the evening to avoid having to get up frequently to use the bathroom.
	Reduce or eliminate caffeinated beverages after noon. Caffeine is a stimulant.
	Reduce or eliminate nicotine after 5 p.m. Nicotine is a stimulant.
	Reduce or eliminate alcohol.
	Avoid bright artificial light (overhead lights, screens) in the two hours before bedtime.
	Use programs on your phone and on your computer to filter out blue spectrum light at night (examples include redshift software, SunsetScreen, CareUEyes, Night Shift, f.lux).
	Get daily exercise but plan to finish at least four hours before bedtime.
	Get up at the same time every morning.
	Keep a consistent bedtime.

After reviewing this list, what are one or two sleep tips that you would like to implement in your life this week?

_____

_____

What are some strategies you plan to use to implement these changes? If you are not sure how to implement these changes, consider revisiting the goal-setting exercise in chapter 6.

_____

_____

_____

_____

EXERCISE 8.3 The Most Important Behavior for Sleep

The *most important* behavior for ensuring good-quality sleep is *getting up at the same time every day*. Wake-up time provides critically important cues for biologic clocks, allowing cortisol levels to rise and starting the build-up of sleep drive that will contribute to good-quality sleep the following night. Below are behaviors and activities that may interfere with getting up regularly at the same time every day. In the spaces provided, describe how these behaviors make it hard for you to maintain a regular wake-up time and what you might do to address the problem. If a behavior does not apply to you, leave it blank. An example is provided to get you started. Blank lines are included at the end for you to add other behaviors that affect the regularity of your wake-up time.

Behavior/Activity	Wake-Up Time Challenges	Possible Solutions
Sleeping in	When I sleep in, I have trouble falling asleep the next night. I then want to sleep in again the following day.	Set two alarms for myself so I make sure I don't oversleep.

Behavior/Activity	Wake-Up Time Challenges	Possible Solutions
Napping		
Staying up later than usual		
Forgetting to set my alarm		
Not exercising		
Taking my medication later than usual		
Scrolling through social media		
Changing schedules on weekends		
Going on vacations		
Changing clocks (spring and fall)		

Being on a schedule that aligns with your chronotype will make it easier for you to get up consistently at the same time every day. If you're a night owl, being on a regular sleep schedule of 1 a.m. to 9 a.m. will probably be more feasible than constantly forcing yourself to go against your natural circadian rhythms. Since most of us revert to our natural rhythms if we don't have good reasons to get up in the mornings, keeping an "unnatural" schedule during the week will make it doubly hard to stay on track with routines during the weekend. Working with—rather than against—your chronotype will set you up to address sleep problems more successfully.

Anxiety and sleep. Feeling anxious makes it hard to sleep, and many individuals with bipolar disorder also struggle with anxiety. When you feel anxious, your mind races, it's hard to relax, and your body reacts with surges of adrenaline (a fight-or-flight response). None of this is helpful if you're trying to fall asleep! If worries are keeping you up at night, try some of these strategies:

- Spend half an hour before bedtime writing down your worries. In addition to writing down your worries, make notes to yourself about how you'll address your concerns the next day. Putting your thoughts on paper may free up your brain to go to sleep. Tip: Don't do your writing while in bed or you'll associate your bed with worrying.

- Keep a "worry journal" next to your bed. If you can't get everything onto paper before bedtime, allow yourself a few minutes to jot a few things on a pad next to your bed to help clear your mind. Tip: Don't spend a lot of time in bed writing about your worries or your bed will become a place for worrying.

- Listen to calming music. Distract yourself before bed with calming, quiet music.

- Let the worries wash over you. Use "self-talk" to remind yourself that the worries can't hurt you right now. Allow them to be present and don't fight them. Sometimes it's the fight that keeps you awake rather than the thoughts themselves.

- Take care of your body. Anxiety is a mind-body experience. When you worry, you have physical symptoms of agitation or activation; when you're agitated or activated, your brain worries. Engaging in activities that calm your body will also calm your brain. For instance, gentle exercise, soothing music, and warm baths can help reduce physical symptoms of anxiety.

- Limit caffeine intake. Caffeine worsens anxiety. The half-life of caffeine is approximately five hours (the time it takes for half of the caffeine ingested to be eliminated), so drinking caffeinated beverages in the afternoon means that you will still have much of that caffeine in your body at night. Tip: Don't drink caffeine after 12 p.m. (noon).

EXERCISE 8.4 Managing Anxiety and Sleep

In the left-hand column, write down worries that keep you up at night. In the right-hand column, write down strategies that you think will be most effective to help you manage your worries. Choose from the list above or add your own ideas.

Worries	Solutions
I think my boyfriend will dump me.	So that I don't play this worry loop on repeat, I'll distract myself with a podcast before bedtime.
I worry about my kids.	I'll write down my worries before I go to bed and not look at them until the morning. I can't do anything about it tonight.

Napping. Napping is a popular way for people to recharge and refresh themselves if they are feeling sleepy midday. Naps are also used to avoid stressful interactions and unpleasant problems. Some people "get away" with napping—that is, they don't notice any negative effects on their nighttime sleep. For many people, especially those with bipolar disorder, naps diminish nighttime sleep drive, making it harder to fall asleep at bedtime. This contributes to a vicious cycle where napping leads to poor sleep which contributes to daytime fatigue which leads to more naps.

If you're having trouble sleeping, avoid daytime naps. If you've had a night of bad sleep, it's best to "power through it," staying awake until bedtime when you'll hopefully fall asleep more easily. If you can't manage to avoid naps, consider brief power naps (twenty minutes or less). Power naps do not usually interfere with your ability to fall asleep. So, if you must nap:

- Nap only during optimal napping hours—i.e., between 1:00 p.m. and 3:00 p.m.

- Keep naps short (under twenty minutes)

- Set an alarm for yourself so that you don't nap for too long

- Nap in a dark room so that you'll fall asleep faster

EXERCISE 8.5 Avoiding Naps

Here are some activities that you might try instead of napping:

- Eat a light meal

- Drink some coffee (but not too late in the day!)

- Exercise midday

- Take a cold shower

- Take a twenty-minute power nap

- Take a walk with a friend

- Listen to loud music

- Drink ice cold water

From the list above, select three strategies that you would use if you had a bad night of sleep and wanted to avoid napping so that you would be able to fall asleep at night. Add comments about how or why these strategies would help you "power through" the day.

Strategy	How It Would Help Me

Sleep efficiency. Sleep efficiency—that is, matching as closely as possible the duration of time that you're in bed to the time that you're actually asleep—is a key component of good-quality sleep. If you spend a lot of time in your bed staring at the clock or worrying about not sleeping, your sleep will not be very efficient. Ideally, you should only spend as much time in bed as you're sleeping, plus about a half hour to give you time to drift off. Here are some tips to improve your sleep efficiency:

- Don't go to sleep unless you're tired. If you aren't sleepy, there is a good chance that you won't fall asleep quickly. Wait until you feel sleepy to lie down.

- If you wake up in the middle of the night, leave your bed until you're sleepy again. Although brief awakenings in the middle of the night are normal, if you're awake for more than about thirty minutes, consider getting out of bed and doing something soothing (e.g., listen to quiet music) until you're sleepy enough to return to bed. Be sure to avoid exposing yourself to any light source (including screens) brighter than a nightlight so that you don't inadvertently suppress melatonin secretion.

- Don't watch the clock. Staring at the clock when you can't sleep will make you anxious and less likely to fall asleep. Turn clocks or screens away from your bed at night so you can't focus on them.

- Use your bed only for sleep and sex. Reserving your bed for sleep (and sex) will help you associate your bed with sleep rather than wakefulness. If you spend lots of time in bed doing other things, your brain is less likely to automatically associate bed with sleep.

- Stay in bed only for the time that you're asleep. If you're spending ten or more hours in bed, but only sleeping for seven or eight of those hours, consider only spending seven or eight hours in bed, even if that means going to bed later than usual and getting up earlier than usual.

- Separate depression from sleepiness. When you're depressed, you may have low energy, low motivation, and low interest. You may interpret this as a signal to crawl into bed. But these are signs of depression rather than readiness for sleep. As a result, you may go to bed but not be able to sleep. Instead of going to bed early, try to find something else to occupy and sooth you (e.g., call a friend, read a book, watch a movie with blue blocking features turned on, practice mindfulness, etc.)

- Mania may interfere with sleep. If you think that trouble sleeping is the result of getting manic or hypomanic, quiet rest in bed, even while awake, may be better than getting out of bed where risk of becoming too active (e.g., cleaning your house) is too high. If this persists, call your doctor.

EXERCISE 8.6 My "I Can't Sleep" Plan

If you're experiencing trouble staying asleep at night, it's helpful to have a plan to manage middle-of-the-night awakenings. Keeping in mind the principles discussed above, write down what you'll do if you awaken in the middle of the night and can't fall back to sleep. Leave a copy of this plan on your nightstand (visit http://www.newharbinger.com/51246 to download one) to remind yourself of what you will do if this happens.

Here is where I will go: _____

This is what I will do: _____

This is what I will *not* do: _____

This is how I will know when it's time to go back to bed: _____

What else can I do to promote good sleep? Because you have a sensitive body clock, it's important to provide your circadian system with as much information about "when" it is during the day as possible to keep it running smoothly. Leveraging the fact that you have circadian sensors throughout your body, consider doing the following three things as soon as you wake up so that your brain knows that is morning. This will put you on good footing (pun intended) to keep your circadian rhythms, including sleep-wake cycle, running smoothly.

1. Get vertical. Put your feet on the floor and stand up. This allows the blood pressure sensors in your vasculature (blood vessels) to send a message to your brain that you're upright and have started your day.

2. Get sunlight. Open the curtains, take a walk outside, or sit on your porch. The sunlight (even if it's cloudy!) signals the cells in the back of your eyes to tell your body clock that it's daytime. Aim for at least two hours of sun exposure each day.

3. Eat something. Putting food or a beverage into your body helps awaken your gastrointestinal (GI) tract. A glass of water may suffice if you can't face food in the morning, but it's probably even better to put something with a few calories into your system, which starts the digestive juices flowing. The circadian sensors in your GI tract then know that you're once again active and can communicate to your brain that the day has begun.

Can medication help my insomnia? Many people with bipolar disorder wish they had a pill to make them fall asleep more easily, stay asleep during the night, and not wake up earlier than necessary. Medication is essential to the management of bipolar disorder, but sleeping pills are not long-term solutions to sleep problems. Medications for sleep rarely provide lasting relief from insomnia, and long-term use may lead to the need for higher and higher doses as your body gets used to lower doses (develops tolerance).

Medications may help in the short run to help break patterns of poor sleep and provide some relief for those who cannot seem to get much sleep. However, enduring improvements in sleep require changes in sleep-related behaviors, including time out of bed, amount of time in bed, and bedtime routines. Management of sleep problems, especially insomnia, with behavior change rather than medication results in better daytime concentration, memory, mood, and quality of life.[113]

Check with your doctor to see what is right for you. Always ask your doctor before stopping or starting any medication or supplement.

EXERCISE 8.7 Strategies for Getting Out of Bed

For some people with bipolar disorder, the main sleep problem is oversleeping. This may be especially true if you're feeling depressed. Although you may strive to adhere to a regular wake-up time, it may feel impossible to get out of bed. And yet, getting out of bed at a regular time is essential to helping you feel better.

Below are strategies that may help you get out of bed in the mornings, especially when you're feeling depressed. These strategies may also be useful if you're trying to reset your sleep-wake cycle by getting up at a time that is earlier than you're used to. Check all the strategies you might be willing to try. To repeat this exercise, please visit http://www.newharbinger.com/51246 for a blank copy.

- ☐ Set multiple alarms, including "annoying" ones that force you to solve a puzzle or do a math problem before they turn off.

- ☐ Vary the location of your alarms. Put at least one of them far away from your bed.

- ☐ Leave your blinds or curtains open at night so that the morning light wakes you up.

- ☐ Ask a friend or family member to give you a wake-up call.

- ☐ Place encouraging thoughts on a notecard beside your bedside table; read immediately upon awakening.

- ☐ Record and then listen to an audio recording on your phone reminding yourself of reasons to get up.

- ☐ Place water on bedside table before you go to sleep. Upon awakening, splash water on your face or drink it.

- ☐ Place something with a strong smell (e.g., cinnamon) on a table next to bed; inhale upon awakening.

- ☐ Throw off the covers immediately when your alarm goes off.

- ☐ Put your feet on the floor immediately when your alarm goes off.

- ☐ Get up and take a shower, even if you feel groggy.

- ☐ Make plans to do something in morning (e.g., meet a friend, go to a volunteer job, sign up for an exercise class).

- ☐ Get a pet who will "force" you to get up in the morning.

Of the items that you checked, which two are likely to be most helpful to you? Write them down below and in your phone. Also, go "old school" and write them on a notecard to put next to your bed as a reminder. Try them out tomorrow.

1. _____

2. _____

Summary. In this chapter, we discussed strategies to help you sleep better. Useful strategies include getting up at the same time every day, avoiding naps, keeping your bedroom dark and cool, and avoiding alcohol. You also developed plans for times when you can't sleep, including knowing in advance where you can go to sit quietly, in darkness, until you're sleepy. Because oversleeping is very common in bipolar disorder, you chose several strategies to help you get out of bed on mornings when you struggle to get up. If you sleep better, you'll feel better.

The next chapter will focus on planned and unplanned disruptions to routines, including strategies to get back on track quickly if your routines become unstable.

CHAPTER 9

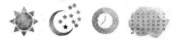

Identifying and Managing Rhythm Disruptors

This chapter will focus on disruptions to routines, both planned and unplanned. Learning to identify and manage potential disruptions to your schedule will help you stay on track with your social rhythms and stabilize your mood.

EXERCISE 9.1 Social Rhythm Metric and Goals Check-In

Your most recent social rhythm goal focused on sleep. Have you noticed connections between your sleep routines and your mood? As you met your sleep goal, did your sleep quality improve? As your sleep improved, did your mood and energy ratings change? Make a few notes below about what you've noticed about your sleep and your moods.

_____

_____

_____

_____

Don't worry if you didn't meet your sleep goal or if your sleep is still not perfect. It can take time to change sleep patterns. Changing sleep schedules is like starting a new exercise routine or stopping smoking: it can be hard at first but usually gets easier if you stick with it. If you're still struggling with sleep problems, revisit chapter 8 to find one strategy that feels manageable and might help your sleep. Maybe it's something as simple as getting some sunshine through a window every morning. Write your new sleep goal below. See if you can hit this goal one or two times this week.

_____

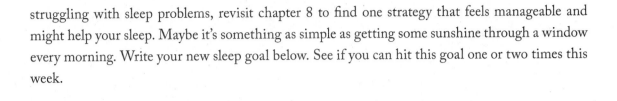

Are you ready to set a new goal? Since we're focusing on rhythm disruptions in this chapter, you might choose minimizing changes to your routines during expected disruptions (e.g., house guests, kids' day off from school, long weekend). This chapter will help you find strategies to meet this goal. Write your new goal(s) here:

_____

_____

_____

What does it mean for you to have a "weak" or sensitive body clock? A weak or sensitive body clock, a common feature of bipolar disorder, means that your internal clock easily loses its rhythm. It shifts from one rhythm to another with relatively minor triggers. From an evolutionary perspective, these types of body clocks enable animals to adapt to challenging environments. For instance, migratory birds with "weak" rhythms adapt more easily to changing light-dark cycles when traveling long distances.[114] Artic animals live with food scarcity; their "weak" rhythms enable them to feed whenever food is available without hunger being tied to specific times of day.[115] For you or your genetic ancestors, this type of flexible body clock may have facilitated adaptation to unpredictable work conditions or food availability. However, for most individuals living today, having sensitive body clocks puts you at odds with the structured environments of work, school, and childcare. It also makes it harder to maintain stable sleep, energy, and appetite routines. When your routines conflict with external schedules (e.g., work times, light-dark schedules, family routines), you're likely to feel badly. Living out of sync with the external world affects your mood.

A sensitive body clock is vulnerable to disruptions caused by environmental changes. For instance, you may find it harder than friends or family members do to recover from jet lag, adapt to daylight savings time, or get back on track after a vacation. Sensitive body clocks rely heavily on external cues to stay in sync with the environment, but today's 24/7, technology-filled world does little to help entrain or synchronize body clocks. Supermarkets and refrigerators provide constant access to food, changing the relationship between food availability and our hunger rhythms. Bright lights interrupt the light-dark cycle that we previously relied upon to re-cue our body clocks each day. If you have a sensitive body clock, you're especially vulnerable to these and other environmental disruptions.

EXERCISE 9.2 Do You Have a Sensitive Body Clock?

If you have bipolar disorder, there is a good chance that you have a sensitive body clock. Below are examples of experiences that may indicate that you have a sensitive body clock. Which scenarios are relevant to your life experience? Check all that apply.

Applies to Me	Rhythm-Disruption Scenarios
	I find it hard to adjust after the clocks change in the spring (to daylight savings time) and fall (to standard time).
	Traveling across time zones leaves me feeling "off" longer than others.
	If I get disturbed during the night, I have trouble falling back to sleep.
	When friends or relatives come stay with me, my schedule gets thrown off for several days.
	If I skip a meal, I never know when I'm going to feel hungry again.
	It's always a struggle for me to get to work on time after the weekend.
	After I stay up late for a night or two, it takes a long time for my bedtime to go back to normal.

Checking one or more of these boxes suggests that your body clock may be extra sensitive to disruptions. Exercises later in this chapter will help you find ways to protect your body clock from disrupting events.

What are zeitstörers? Zeitstörer means "time disturber" in German. Circadian researchers use this term to describe external factors that disturb the body clock. Everyone experiences zeitstörers, or disruptions in their routines. For instance, starting back to school after summer vacation disrupts summer routines. A newborn baby inevitably disturbs its parents' pre-baby routines. Can you think of a time in the last few weeks that your routines were disrupted? What happened in your life and how did it affect your routines?

_____

_____

_____

Common examples of physical or environmental zeitstörers include shifts from daylight savings time to standard time (and vice versa) and medical illnesses that keep you up all night. Social zeitstörers, or social demands or factors that disrupt your body clock, include unexpected house guests, rotating shift work, exams or heavy work demands, new jobs, and retirement. These zeitstörers are, of course, a normal part of life. However, if you have a sensitive body clock, your routines are more likely to be thrown off by these disruptions than for someone whose body clock is less vulnerable.

Technology and social media can also act as zeitstörers. Scrolling endlessly through social media can push back your bedtime, make it harder for you to finish work in the allotted time, or cause you to show up late for an activity or event. Video chats may eat into your exercise time or stop you from getting regular sun exposure. How does technology affect your routines?

_____

_____

_____

EXERCISE 9.3 Identifying Zeitstörers

What are some examples of zeitstörers in your life? Circle the zeitstörers that apply to you. In the space next to the zeitstörer, reflect on the effect that this disrupting factor had or will have on your routines. An example is provided to get you started. There is also space to add additional relevant zeitstörers.

Zeitstörer	Personal Reflections
(A new pet)	When I got a puppy, it kept me up at night with its whining. I also had to get used to taking it outside for walks twice a day.

Zeitstörer	Personal Reflections
Travel across time zones	
Social media	
Vacation	
Final exams	
COVID pandemic	
New job	
Unemployment	
Divorce	
New romantic partner	
Moving	
Surgery	
Childcare/new baby	

Managing planned and unplanned disruptions. Some rhythm disruptions are anticipated or planned (e.g., vacations, invited guests, switch to daylight savings time); others are unplanned (e.g., trips to the emergency room, unexpected houseguests, natural disasters). Although both planned and unplanned zeitstörers can affect your body clock, strategies to manage these events' impact on routines are somewhat different.

When a zeitstörer is anticipated, it's helpful to do some planning in advance to figure out how to handle those disruptions in such a way as to minimize their impact on your body clock.

For instance, if you're expecting to travel across several time zones, you can gradually (over a week or two) *shift your schedule a little earlier or later* (depending on the direction of your travel) so that there is less of a difference between the time at home and the time at your destination. The smaller the gap between the time at home and the time at your destination, the easier it is to manage jet lag. If you anticipate that some aspects of your schedule will change (for example, changes in sleep-wake times while on a vacation), *try keeping other parts of your schedule regular.* For instance, try to eat meals and exercise at your usual times. Another helpful strategy is to *ask for help*. For instance, you could speak to your houseguests before their arrival, explain your schedule to them, and ask that they stay on your schedule while visiting. You could work with a disability officer at school to stagger your exams so that you don't have to radically alter your schedule at the end of the semester. Mothers of newborns can protect their sleep by asking their partner or a supportive family member to give the baby a bottle for nighttime feeding. These strategies will help alleviate the circadian challenges associated with disrupting events and keep your body clock running smoothly.

When a disruption is unplanned (e.g., emergency room visit, last minute work deadline), the focus should be *reestablishing regular routines as quickly as possible* after the disruption. For instance, following a night of decreased sleep, try to stay awake during the day (without napping) and do your usual activities. Even if you feel tired, staying on your usual schedule (including waiting until your usual bedtime to go to sleep) will help you get back on track quickly. If you must nap, take a brief (twenty-minute) power nap relatively early in the day so that you don't have trouble falling asleep. Below are some tips for managing rhythm disruptions:

- Get back on your schedule. Restart your old schedule as soon as possible after a break. If you spend the night in an emergency room, for instance, you may need to take a brief nap the next day but try to go to bed at your usual time. Get up the following day at the usual time so your body clock can reset itself.

- Use light to reset your clock. Remember that exposure to light in the morning can help your clock reset itself. For instance, if you have unexpected house guests who keep you up later than usual, invite them to take a walk with you in the morning to get your daytime schedule off to a good start.

- Stick to your old schedule. When you have a change in your routines, try to recreate your old schedule for yourself. If you lose your job or go on vacation, put activities in place that keep you busy during times that would normally have been busy on your old schedule.

- Keep part of your schedule in place. If your life is thrown into chaos (newborn, family illness, travel), try to stick to at least part of your schedule. For instance, even if your sleep schedule is off, try to keep your meal schedule in place. Or vice versa.

- Manage your technology. To avoid technology-related rhythm disruptions, turn off your devices at least an hour before bedtime, consider installing an app on electronic devices to limit the amount of blue light exposure at night (see chapter 8), and limit your social media use, especially at night.

EXERCISE 9.4 Managing Rhythm-Disrupting Events

Select a zeitstörer from exercise 9.3 that recently affected your routines or will cause disruptions in the future. Describe the disrupting event here:

_____

How did/will this event affect your routines? Your mood?

_____

_____

Is this event planned or unplanned? _____

Is there anything you will do or could have done to keep your routines regular in the face of the zeitstörer? List ideas here:

_____

_____

_____

Below are some suggestions for managing rhythm disruptions. Circle strategies that you might consider using to address this or other disruptions. In the column next to the strategy, explain how you would implement it. An example is provided to get you started. There are blank spaces at the end for you to add more ideas.

Strategy	What I Will Do
Keep some routines in place even when others are changing.	I'll continue to eat dinner at 7 p.m. while I am on vacation, even though I'll be on a later schedule.
Take steps to minimize the impact of the disruption on my routines.	
Look ahead in my calendar to identify potential disruptions.	
Make gradual changes before the event to move my routines closer to those at my upcoming destination.	
Ask for help to minimize disruptions.	
Use a calendar to figure out when disruptions may occur and plan for them	
Get back on track as soon as possible.	
Get up at the same time each day—even if my other routines are shifted.	
Monitor my social media use to make sure it isn't affecting routines.	

Summary. In this chapter, you learned to identify and anticipate zeitstörers, including planned and unplanned disruptions to routines. You developed strategies to address rhythm disruptions, including asking for help and getting back on track as quickly as possible if your routines become unstable.

In the next chapter, we'll explore the rhythm disrupting and stabilizing effects of relationships. You'll be encouraged to examine how some people and interactions in your life help your routines stay on track while others disrupt your routines. We'll discuss strategies to address relationship challenges that contribute to social rhythm disruptions.

CHAPTER 10

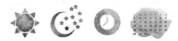

Relationships and Rhythms

This chapter discusses the impact that relationships can have on rhythms and mood. Some relationships help stabilize moods by helping us stay on track with our routines; other relationships disrupt routines. By understanding how relationships both help and hurt routines and mood, you'll become familiar with additional strategies you can use to stabilize your social rhythms and thereby stabilize your mood.

EXERCISE 10.1 Social Rhythm Goals Check-In

Record your reflections below about recent experiences working toward a social rhythm goal. Did you identify a planned or unplanned zeitstörer in your life? Did you notice connections between the zeitstörer and the regularity of your SRM? Between the regularity of your SRM and your mood? What strategies did you use to get back on track?

_____

_____

_____

Did you recently meet a social rhythm goal? If so, congratulations! Note below what you have accomplished so far.

_____

_____

Not everyone will have achieved their social rhythm goals. As you work toward rhythm regularity, it's not uncommon to take one step forward and then one step back. If you haven't yet met your goal(s), you're not alone. It can be helpful, however, to think about what stands in your way. What barriers have you encountered as you try to move forward with your goals?

_____

_____

What are some strategies you might try in the upcoming days to address those barriers? (Hints: Break the goal into smaller pieces; reward yourself for taking steps toward regularity; be gentle with yourself if you're not yet ready to move forward.)

_____

_____

What social rhythm goal would you like to work on next? If you're still struggling to meet earlier goals, it's fine to select a previous goal (or, even better, a less ambitious but perhaps more attainable version of an earlier goal). If you're ready to pick a new goal, perhaps choose one at the intersection of your relationships and your social rhythms. For instance, you could invite a friend to go walking with you in the mornings if you're having trouble meeting your exercise or first contact goal (or both). Write your goal down here:

_____

People and moods. Humans are social creatures, and our moods are strongly influenced by the people around us. Better quality relationships help us feel better[116] and loneliness contributes to depression and poor health outcomes.[117] Not all relationships affect us equally, however. Some relationships are protective, buffering us from life's stresses,[118] whereas others cause social strain,[119] potentially making us feel worse. When you have bipolar disorder, it's important to consider how relationships affect your mood.

EXERCISE 10.2 RELATIONSHIPS AND MOOD

Identify a close relationship, for instance, a romantic partner, child, parent, sibling, coworker, or friend. Think about this person as you respond to the prompts below.

When I'm with _____, I usually feel (select all that apply):

☐ Happy	☐ Unsafe	☐ Excited
☐ Sad	☐ Joyful	☐ Stressed
☐ Anxious	☐ Relaxed	☐ Relieved
☐ Safe	☐ Bored	☐ _____

Reflect on the combination of feelings that you checked in the list above. Most people have both positive and negative feelings about relationships.

What are some positive aspects of this relationship?

_____

What are some negative aspects of this relationship?

_____

How does your relationship affect your mood and your bipolar disorder?

_____

The next exercise will help you think about ways to improve your relationships, thereby enhancing your mood.

EXERCISE 10.3 Improving Relationships

Thinking about the relationship you identified in exercise 10.2 (or another relationship, if you prefer), respond to the following prompts.

What would you like to change about this relationship?

_____

How would these changes affect your mood stability?

_____

_____

Below is a list of strategies to improve relationships. Check all that might be helpful to your relationship.

☐ Spend more time together in person (versus online).

☐ Make direct, positive requests when speaking with the other person. Direct requests, devoid of insults or criticism, can make it easier to negotiate or handle disagreements. Here is an example: "Please let me finish telling you about my concerns before responding. I'll be better able to hear your feedback if I express how I feel without interruption."

☐ If you disagree, discuss it in person rather than by sending text messages. Text messages are often misinterpreted because the reader lacks other important contextual cues, such as facial expression, tone of voice, and body language.

☐ Express gratitude for the other person. Let them know why you value them.

☐ Set limits. Be very clear about what you will and will not do with or for the other person. It's okay to say, "I really care about you, but I cannot drive you to your job at 4 a.m. every day. These early morning rides are negatively affecting my health."

☐ Schedule a time to talk about difficult issues when both parties are calm rather than when one or both of you are upset. If both of you are clear-headed, you're more likely to find constructive solutions.

☐ Set differences aside for a few hours and do something fun together.

☐ Ask a neutral third party (e.g., clergyman, therapist, trusted advisor) to help negotiate solutions to difficult problems in the relationship.

☐ Express contrition for your contributions to misunderstandings or disagreements before asking for an apology.

☐ Accept that some things can't be changed. If you have tried to make changes, worked with a therapist or clergy to try to improve the situation, and engaged in constructive discussions, it may be time to adjust your expectations. Accepting that someone can't change is hard, but it may free you up to focus your energies elsewhere.

☐ Agree to disagree and move on.

Which of these strategies might you implement this week? Describe how and when you're going to give it try.

_____

_____

_____

How do you think these strategies will affect your emotions and mood?

_____

_____

_____

_____

Problematic communication styles. Effective communication is necessary to convey your needs or wishes to others in your life. If you want to ask for help in keeping your rhythms on track, you need to find ways to do so effectively. When you have bipolar disorder, your symptoms can negatively impact your communication patterns—for instance, irritability can push people away or depression can make it hard to muster the energy to engage others in conversation. Therefore, it's important to be mindful of ways that communication can go awry. Here are examples of problematic communication behaviors:

- Yelling, shouting, raising your voice
- Teasing or making fun of the other person
- Threatening the other person
- Ignoring the other person's ideas or requests
- Interrupting a lot
- Blaming the other person
- Talking very little or remaining silent
- Using put-downs or criticisms

- Using a sarcastic tone of voice

- Swearing or cursing

- Thinking that you know best

- Walking out or turning your back on the conversation

We all use ineffective communication strategies some of the time. If you have bipolar disorder, you may notice that you use these strategies more often when feeling depressed or manic. Becoming aware of when and why you use these problematic communication patterns can help you improve them and, most likely, improve your relationships.

EXERCISE 10.4 Managing Problematic Communication

Managing challenging interpersonal relationships is a complicated business. Working with a therapist is probably the best way to learn how to effectively navigate relationship dynamics; however, you can also independently consider communication behaviors that may contribute to or help address problematic interactions. This exercise is intended to help you think about some of these behaviors. If you are working with a therapist, consider sharing these reflections with her.

Which problematic communications strategies do you use? How has this affected your relationships?

_____

Which problematic communication strategies do you use when feeling *depressed*? How has this affected your relationships?

_____

Which problematic communication strategies do you use when feeling *hypomanic or manic*? How has this affected your relationships?

_____

Below are examples of strategies you might use to improve problematic communications. Check whether the strategies would be most helpful to you when you're depressed, hypo/manic, or stable. If the strategy would be helpful in more than one mood state, check all that apply.

- Set the stage for effective communication. Make sure your surroundings are optimal for having the conversation that you hope to have. Turn off the TV, turn down the music, make sure the kids are not underfoot, turn off your phones. Sit where you can see each other, hear each other, and talk uninterrupted.

   (This strategy could be helpful when I am   ☐ depressed   ☐ manic or hypomanic   ☐ stable.)

- State your needs clearly. Make sure you know what you want to say so that you can say it clearly to the other person. Ask yourself these questions before starting the conversation.

   - What are your goals?

   - What do you want to get out of the discussion?

   - What do you want the other person to understand about your point of view?

   - Do you plan to make a request?

   - What do you hope will be the outcome of the communication?

   (This strategy could be helpful when I am   ☐ depressed   ☐ manic or hypomanic   ☐ stable.)

- Use "I" statements. "I" statements focus on the feelings of the speaker rather than opinions about the other person's motives, feelings, or intent. For instance, instead of saying, "*You* really piss me off when you go off and do things without me," try saying, "*I* feel hurt when you go out with other friends and don't include me. *I* would appreciate it if you would try to include me too." Moving from "you" to "I" may make the listener feel less defensive and therefore more receptive to your concerns.

   (This strategy could be helpful when I am   ☐ depressed   ☐ manic or hypomanic   ☐ stable.)

- Be a good listener. Listening is at least as important as talking. Learn to be a better listener. Try some of these strategies to improve your listening skills:

   - *Listen* to the person speaking, rather than the "noise" around you.

   - *Look* at the speaker directly, making eye contact.

   - Nod and use *encouraging statements* like "uh huh" to show that you're listening.

- Reflect what is said back to the speaker by *paraphrasing* their main points.

- *Ask questions* to get clarification.

- *Don't look at your text messages or phone while you're talking.*

(This strategy could be helpful when I am   ☐ depressed   ☐ manic or hypomanic
☐ stable.)

- Assert yourself. Be assertive in conversations, not aggressive. Respect the feelings and opinions of others but also advocate for yourself. Here are some strategies you might use to effectively assert yourself:

  - Speak firmly and clearly.

  - State your needs and wishes directly, without drama but with clarity.

  - Express your feelings but don't be too emotional.

  - Practice or rehearse what you want to say before saying it.

(This strategy could be helpful when I am   ☐ depressed   ☐ manic or hypomanic
☐ stable.)

- Explain yourself. Especially when feeling depressed, you may not have the energy or concentration needed to express yourself well. Although this is understandable, it has a negative effect on relationships. Explaining how you're feeling and why you're behaving this way can help your relationships.

  - Explain what happens to your mood and energy when you're in an episode.

  - Apologize in advance (or retrospectively) for not being a good communicator during these periods.

  - Explain to the other person or people how they can be helpful to you when you feel depressed or manic.

  - Explain what is *not* helpful when you feel this way.

  - Consider some strategies that you might be able to use to improve communication even when you feel badly such as carving out time for conversations or asking for help or support. Write yourself a note to remind yourself how you would like to handle communication when feeling depressed, anxious, or hypomanic.

(This strategy could be helpful when I am   ☐ depressed   ☐ manic or hypomanic   ☐ stable.)

As with most skills, practice is required to achieve mastery. Depending on how you're feeling right now, which strategy would you like to try practicing first?

_____

How might this strategy help you better manage a challenging relationship problem?

_____

When, where, and with whom will you use the skill?

_____

_____

Learning new skills is hard. What are some challenges you anticipate as you practice this new communication skill?

_____

_____

_____

How will your bipolar disorder impact your ability to use or practice this skill?

_____

If or when you run into barriers practicing the skill, how might you overcome the barrier? (Hint: First, practice with yourself in the mirror; ask a trusted friend or relative to practice the skill with you; practice the skill on paper as a written exercise before test-driving it with a real person.)

_____

_____

_____

Relationships and rhythms. In addition to impacting our well-being directly, relationships indirectly affect our mood by affecting our circadian rhythms.[120] In fact, the main rationale for SRT is that social factors, including relationships, help to entrain our circadian rhythms,[121] thereby helping to stabilize mood.

Relationships serve as social rhythm anchors, or zeitgebers. For instance, parents are awakened by young children, thereby shaping sleep schedules. The day begins with greetings to flat mates or the barista making our coffees, creating consistent first contacts for the day. Partners prepare meals for each other, and roommates help each other wind down in the evening, thereby stabilizing meal-times and bedtimes. These social ties, both weak and strong, help to organize the rhythms of our days.

Relationships can also act as social rhythm disrupters, or zeitstörers. For instance, when children are on summer vacation or have an unexpected day off, parents' schedules are thrown into disarray. When friends cancel plans, it may be harder to follow through with scheduled activities, like workouts or leisure activities. Online companions may encourage us to use our screens late at night, increasing blue spectrum light exposure and suppressing melatonin production. Romantic partners who fight with us late into the evening may disrupt sleep schedules and routines. Thus, body clocks are strongly influenced by the people in our lives—both those who help keep our schedules running smoothly and those who get it off on track.

EXERCISE 10.5 Relationships and Rhythms

Think about your relationships, both those that serve as anchors and those that cause disruptions (sometimes the same person can do both!). Keep these relationships in mind as you complete the following exercise.

Here is an example of a relationship that keeps my rhythms on track:

_____

Here is how they help keep my routines stable: _____

_____

They affect my mood or bipolar disorder in the following ways: _____

_____

I'll use these communication strategies to express my appreciation for their help with my social rhythms:

_____

Here is an example of a relationship that destabilizes my rhythms: _____

_____

Here is how they help disrupt my routines: _____

_____

They affect my mood or bipolar disorder in the following ways: _____

_____

I'll use these communication strategies to request changes to better protect my social rhythms:

_____

EXERCISE 10.6 Stabilizing Relationships

In chapter 9, you learned about strategies to manage social rhythm disruptions. Most of these strategies can also apply to managing the social rhythm aspects of disrupting relationships, with some modifications or additions. Below are strategies that you can use to lessen the negative effects of rhythm-disrupting relationships. After each example, there is space for you to write down how these strategies might apply in your life. Consider whether each approach would be most helpful to you when you're in a depressed, hypomanic, or stable mood.

- Ask the people in your life to help you stabilize your routines. For instance, let friends know that it's very helpful for your social rhythms to schedule morning walks or coffee dates. Ask them if they would be willing to put some regular meetings on the calendar. Use some of the communication skills discussed above to effectively request help.

    This approach would be helpful to me in the following circumstance(s):

    _____

- Limit screen time and blue light exposure. Especially for relationships that take place primarily online, make sure that you consider the time of day that you interact virtually with your friend, partner, or colleague. Limit blue spectrum light from screens at night. Consider asking the individual to meet earlier in the day or use technology fixes to decrease blue spectrum light exposure.

  This approach would be helpful to me in the following circumstance(s):

  _____

- Fight at the right time. Arguing activates the flight-or-fight response, flooding the body with activating hormones. If you fight at night, it makes it hard to settle down and fall asleep. If you're in a contentious relationship where you engage in vigorous disagreements late at night, speak with your partner or friend about changing the time of day that you have these disputes. Schedule the discussion for a weekend day or earlier in the evening. Don't fight at night.

  This approach would be helpful to me in the following circumstance(s):

  _____

- Get back on track as soon as possible. If you have experienced a relationship-related disruption, try to get back on track with your routines as soon as possible. Following a break-up, reach out to friends to schedule meals and activities to take the place of your ex-partner's social prompts. After staying up all night with a sick child, keep yourself busy and avoid naps so that you can get back on your normal sleep schedule that night.

  This approach would be helpful to me in the following circumstance(s):

  _____

- Talk about it. If someone in your life is disrupting your social rhythms, let them know. Explain to them the concepts of social anchors and disturbers (maybe share this book with them!). Ask them if they might be willing to support your goals. Think about the communication skills outlined above to help you navigate your discussion. Take time before the discussion to make a list of your needs and wishes.

  This approach would be helpful to me in the following circumstance(s):

  _____

EXERCISE 10.7 Addressing Disrupting Relationships

In the left column, identify instances when relationships have disrupted your routines. In the right column, write down strategies that you might use to manage the disruption. You can select a technique from the lists in the preceding sections or add your own ideas. An example is provided.

How the Relationship Affects My Routines	How I Can Address This Disruption
Steven and I always fight about the kids and chores after the kids have gone to bed...about who is going to pick them up from school, who is going to the laundry. After we fight, I have a hard time going to sleep, which throws my schedule off for the next day.	I'll make a list of chores/childcare responsibilities that need to be divided between us for the week. I'll ask Steven to carve out time on Saturday while his parents are watching the kids to figure out the schedule for the week. I'll explain to him why I don't want to get into it at night.

How the Relationship Affects My Routines	How I Can Address This Disruption

Regular rhythms are good for everyone. As discussed previously (chapter 7), disrupted routines are detrimental to most individuals, increasing risk of numerous problems including mood episodes, cardiovascular disease, diabetes, obesity, and even some cancers.[122] Conversely, regular routines are helpful for most of us.

Try engaging your friends, family, and social support network in your pursuit of social rhythm regularity. Explain to them why circadian and social rhythms are important. Invite them to accompany you on your social rhythm regularity journey. Show them this book. It will be easier for you to stay on a regular routine if the important people in your life share or at least understand your quest for social rhythm regularity. This situation is not unlike trying to lose weight: if you're trying to eat healthily or lose weight, you can certainly work on it by yourself, but you're more likely to be successful if those around you are also trying to eat healthily. Even if they are not trying to lose weight, they, too, will probably feel better if they follow a healthy diet. Similarly, most people in your social network will feel better with regular social rhythms, even if they don't have bipolar disorder.

If you anticipate a big disruption in your household routines (vacation, holidays, visitors), get everyone involved in sticking to a regular routine. Put up a big calendar or dry erase board in a common space where you can write down times for meals and scheduled events. If you can get everyone to follow a schedule, it will help you stay on track—and it will help them too.

Here's what I will do to get others involved in my journey toward having more regular routines:

_____

_____

Summary. In this chapter, you learned about the links among relationships, rhythms, and mood. You learned that some relationships help with mood and rhythm stability while others disrupt them. You extended your repertoire of strategies to address rhythm disruptions by learning new ways to address relationship behaviors that interfere with rhythm stability. You considered effective strategies for communication and ways to engage your social network in supporting your social rhythm stability.

In the next and final chapter, you'll look at how far you have come in your journey to achieve regular routines and rhythms. We'll discuss strategies to prevent mood episode in the future, with special attention to the role of SRM monitoring to prevent episode recurrences. We'll wrap up with suggestions on how to continue SRT work in the future.

CHAPTER 11

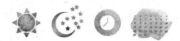

Relapse Prevention and Rhythms

This final chapter provides you with an opportunity to reflect on progress made in stabilizing your social rhythms and its impact on your mood. It will conclude with rhythm-focused strategies that you can use to maintain wellness.

EXERCISE 11.1 Assessing Progress

As this book comes to an end, think about what you have accomplished since beginning this workbook. Below are some questions that you were asked to consider in exercise 7.1 (and can also be found at http://www.newharbinger.com/51246). After answering the same questions again, you'll be encouraged to compare the two sets of responses to see how far you have come.

To assess your SRT progress, rate the extent to which you agree with the following statements:

I have increased the regularity of my daily routines.

Strongly Agree_____   Agree_____   Undecided_____   Disagree_____   Strongly Disagree_____

I can identify the symptoms of bipolar disorder.

Strongly Agree_____   Agree_____   Undecided_____   Disagree_____   Strongly Disagree_____

I know how to evaluate my SRMs.

Strongly Agree_____   Agree_____   Undecided_____   Disagree_____   Strongly Disagree_____

I feel comfortable rating my mood on a –5 to +5 scale.

Strongly Agree_____   Agree_____   Undecided_____   Disagree_____   Strongly Disagree_____

I have successfully completed at least one social rhythm goal.

Strongly Agree_____   Agree_____   Undecided_____   Disagree_____   Strongly Disagree_____

I recognize the link between daily rhythms and moods in my own life.

Strongly Agree_____   Agree_____   Undecided_____   Disagree_____   Strongly Disagree_____

I can identify *stabilizing* social rhythm anchors in my life.

Strongly Agree_____   Agree_____   Undecided_____   Disagree_____   Strongly Disagree_____

I can recognize and anticipate *disrupting* social rhythm factors in my life.

Strongly Agree_____   Agree_____   Undecided_____   Disagree_____   Strongly Disagree_____

I can get my life back on track after a social rhythm disruption.

Strongly Agree_____   Agree_____   Undecided_____   Disagree_____   Strongly Disagree_____

I have very regular daily routines.

Strongly Agree_____   Agree_____   Undecided_____   Disagree_____   Strongly Disagree_____

For which items did you choose "strongly agree" or "agree"? Compare your responses above to your answers in chapter 7. Are any of these different compared to chapter 7? Note these items below:

_____

_____

These are probably areas where you have made a lot of progress in SRT, either before or since you worked on chapter 7. Congratulations on your accomplishments!

For which items did you answer "undecided" or "disagree" or "strongly disagree"? Are any of these different compared to chapter 7? Note these items below:

_____

_____

These are areas that you're probably still working on. Even though you're coming to the end of the book, it's normal to feel like you have not mastered all components of SRT or that you are backsliding in some areas. Establishing and maintaining stable social rhythms are self-care practices that you'll hopefully continue to explore, even after finishing this book. As you continue to work on rhythm regularity, you might find it helpful to consider some of the strategies listed below:

- Revisit information contained in earlier chapters. For ease of reference, there are brief summaries of topics covered at the beginning of each chapter. You can flip through the book to look for topics that you would like to work on, returning to those chapters as needed. Repetition is a good way to achieve mastery.

- Revisit your social rhythm goals. Look back through the book to identify prior goals. Which ones continue to be challenging? Can you select from your prior goals one that you would like to revisit now, having finished most of the book? As you learn more skills, you might find it easier to achieve your goals.

- Be an SRM detective. Your increased understanding of factors affecting social rhythms enables you to take a more nuanced view of your SRMs. Revisit old SRMs to find hitherto undiscovered links between regularity and mood. Rather than looking at a single SRM, look at several consecutive weeks of SRMs to find patterns over time. Are you consistently struggling during the week? The weekend? Is there variability in your mood related to identified zeitstörers? How are your relationships affecting these patterns? Revisiting your SRMs may help you better discern—and then address—problematic patterns in your social rhythms.

- Break your goals into smaller pieces. As always, if you struggle to meet your social rhythm goals, break them into smaller pieces. Build slowly and gradually on small accomplishments.

- Involve others. Talk with friends and family about how they can help you to achieve rhythm regularity. Get them interested in working on SRT with you. Set shared goals for your social rhythms and then compare notes on progress toward meeting goals.

- Be gentle with yourself. When you live with bipolar disorder, moods can be unpredictable. If you're having a bad week, set even more modest goals for yourself. If you backslide, be kind to yourself, acknowledging that progress is rarely steady or linear. Don't give up, but don't hold yourself to unattainable goals. As the saying goes, slow and steady wins the race.

Relapse prevention. Catching mood episodes early may allow you to head them off. Many people notice that one specific symptom (or more) routinely occurs before a full mood episode sets in. We call these "early warning signs." The time between these first symptoms and "full-blown" mania or depression is different for every person. Early warning signs can last anywhere from a day to several weeks. You can train yourself to recognize them, buying yourself time to address them before they become too problematic.

In practice, warning signs may be hard to detect in daily life. Symptoms are often mild and don't cause major problems. To identify your personal warning signs, think about your last depressive or manic episode. What symptoms do you remember starting first? Sometimes friends and family members notice changes before you do, so check in with them. What do they remember? What does your doctor or therapist say? By thinking about your own experiences and querying the observations of others, you can get better at recognizing your early warning signs.

Relapse prevention planning involves identifying early warning signs and deciding in advance actions to take when they start. *In the next exercise, you'll think about your own episode triggers and early warning signs.*

EXERCISE 11.2 Mood Episode Triggers

Think back to what was going on in your life just before the start of a recent depressive or manic episode in your life. What kinds of changes happened before your mood shifted? Below are common triggering activities. Check any that apply to you. In the space provided, make notes reflecting on the relationship between the triggering event and your social rhythms. Spaces are left at the end for you to write about additional triggers.

This Applies to Me	Trigger	How the Trigger Affected My Social Rhythms
	More pressure/demands at work or home	
	Staying up most of the night to care for a sick relative/friend	
	Exams or big work deadlines	
	Skipping medications	
	Vacation or travel	
	Changing or losing a job	
	Physical illness	
	Retirement	
	Moving	
	New romantic relationship	
	Ending a romantic relationship	
	Entering/leaving military service	

	Death of an important person in your life	
	Microaggressions/racism	
	Trauma	

By identifying stressors that have triggered episodes in the past, you can develop strategies to manage them more effectively in the future. For instance, if you developed your first manic episode after an especially difficult exam period in college, you may be vulnerable to developing mood episodes in the context of high stress situations and sleep deprivation. You may wish to identify future potentially stressful events and decide to be especially vigilant about your routines—including sleep, eating, and exercise—before, during, and after the event.

What potential triggering events are likely to occur in the future?

_____

How will the triggering event affect your social rhythms?

_____

If you experience this event, what could you do to prevent it from disrupting your social rhythms?

_____

EXERCISE 11.3 Early Warning Signs

Below is a list of possible early warning signs. Check the items that you're likely to experience or notice before a hypomanic or manic episode and those that you're likely to experience before a depressive episode. If you're not sure, ask friends and family who were involved in your life at the time what they recall.

Note that some warning signs may precede either mania or depression. For example, increased irritability and anxiety could be a warning sign for mania in one person and a warning sign for depression in another person. Warning signs that are common for mania *and* depression include:

- Insomnia

- Anxiety

- Poor concentration

- Irritability

For the warning signs below, check which ones are relevant to you. You can also make notes in the box to indicate how this specifically occurs for you. For instance, if very minor insomnia precedes hypomania, you might indicate that you should pay attention if your sleep decreases by thirty to forty minutes a night. If a warning sign precedes both mania and depression, mark both boxes. There is space at the end for you to add additional personalized warning signs.

Early Warning Sign	Precedes Hypomania/ Mania	Precedes Depression
Talking faster and louder		
Invading other people's personal space		
Needing less sleep		
Oversleeping		
Feeling more anxious		
Making impulsive decisions		
Starting lots of new activities		
Feeling slowed down/fatigued		
Feeling numb		
Being irritable or snappy		
Being more self-critical		
Feeling hopeless		
Lower self esteem		
Loss of interest in things you usually like		
Withdrawing from people you normally talk to		

What should I do if I notice early warning signs? Here are some tips to help navigate early warning signs.

- Don't panic. Ups and downs are part of life. Just because you're feeling worse, it may not mean that you're starting to get depressed or manic. You may be having a bad day. If the early warning sign persists for several days, however, you may wish to address it.

- Use your SRMs to get back on track. If you get in the habit of monitoring your mood and daily rhythms regularly, you may notice changes before they get out of control. Tracking mood and rhythm changes will give you a chance to put a relapse prevention plan into place early (more about creating such a plan below).

- Focus on your rhythms. If you notice that you're feeling worse, double down on your routines and rhythms. Take a few days to focus on keeping "supranormal rhythms" in most areas of your life. Track your mood to see if it improves as you resume or strengthen regular routines.

- Ask other people for help. Getting help from others does not take away from all that you have accomplished. It shows that you have learned to take advantage of your social support network. Ask for help if you need it.

- Remember that it's not your fault. Worsening mood may indicate that this self-help approach is not for you or that you need more help in managing your bipolar disorder than self-help can provide. Or, it may reflect the natural ebb and flow of your bipolar disorder. Talk to your doctor about treatment options.

- Don't forget about the emergency room. If things get really bad or you're in crisis, you can always go to the nearest emergency room. Emergency rooms are set up to provide you with care right away. If you are thinking about suicide, call or text (in the US) 988, which is the National Suicide Prevention Line.

- Seek outpatient mental health services. If you do not already see a psychiatrist or other prescriber, speak with your primary care doctor or insurance provider about treatment options; they will be able to connect you with behavioral health prescribers in your community. To find a therapist, consider checking out the Psychology Today website, which maintains rosters of therapists, sorted by location. Low-fee psychotherapy options can be found at http://www.healwise.org.

EXERCISE 11.4 Who Can Help?

Who might you wish to ask for help if you're having a hard time? In the exercise below, you'll be asked to list individuals whom you might approach during setbacks or mood symptom flare-ups. For each individual, list the pros and cons of including them in your relapse prevention plan. For instance, perhaps you trust a coworker to drop everything to help you but worry they might talk about you at work. Perhaps you're sure that your mother would always be there for you but you're worried about burdening her because of her declining health. Listing pros and cons can help you decide whom you're willing to contact if you need help. On the far right, list the kinds of things you would ask this specific person to help you with. For example, you might request help with dog-walking, grocery shopping, meal preparation, social rhythm regularity, or emotional support. An example is provided to get you started.

Person	Pros	Cons	What I Will Ask of Them
Sister	Always wants to help	Puts her nose in my business	Pick up groceries, help me figure out what to tell my boss, remind me to shower

Once you have decided whom you would like to include on your list, it's important that you ask their permission to contact them should you need it. It can be helpful to plan out what you'll say to them when you ask. Here is an example of what you might say:

As you know, I have bipolar disorder. I am trying to develop a plan to help myself manage better when I start to have mood symptoms. As part of my plan, I am identifying people I can call if I am having a hard time. Is it okay if I reach out to you if I need help? For instance, I might ask you to take a walk with me if I am feeling depressed or give me a ride to the doctor's office if I don't feel up to managing public transportation. If this is not feasible for you, I understand. If this is okay with you, however, would you prefer me to text you, call you, or stop by? Also, when I am getting sick, I am usually stuck in my own head and am not able to express gratitude, so I want to say in advance that I truly appreciate your friendship, love, and support.

Write out what you will say to friends or family when you ask them to support you if needed. After writing it down, practice saying it out loud to yourself in the mirror once or twice if you're worried about how it will go.

_____

_____

_____

_____

_____

EXERCISE 11.5 Personalized Relapse Prevention Plan

In this exercise, you'll create a personalized relapse prevention plan. This plan can be used to help you monitor your early warning signs and, in an easily accessible way, tell yourself what you should do if you notice something is going awry. You can also find a copy to download and print at http://www.newharbinger.com/51246.

For each warning sign, write down what you're likely to notice early in a depressive episode and early in a manic episode. For instance, for sleep, you might note that it's likely to increase when you start to get depressed and decrease when you start to get manic. If an item does not apply to you, leave it blank. Review exercise 11.3 to remind yourself of your previously identified early warning signs. In the right column, add information about whom you'll contact, what you would like them to do for you, how you'll modify your daily routines to get back on track, and what would trigger you to call your doctor. After completing this relapse prevention plan, give copies to friends and family members.

Warning Sign	Depression	(Hypo)mania	Relapse Prevention Plan Action
Anger level			If I notice early warning signs, I will contact these individuals: 1. 2.
Sleep			If I contact a support person, I would like them to: 1. 2.
Appetite			
Energy			If I notice changes in my daily routines, I will increase regularity of my routines by doing the following: 1. 2.
Concentration			
Interest in activities			I will use these relapse prevention strategies (check all that apply): ☐ Double down on tracking SRMs ☐ Pay more attention to regularity of routines
Interest in sex			☐ Get more sleep ☐ Add more activities/keep busy
Ability to make decisions			☐ Ask a friend or relative to help monitor my mood and behavior
Level of worry/ anxiety			☐ Call my doctor Phone numbers for my doctor and therapist:
Other signs (specify)			1. 2.

You're on a path to success! Congratulations on completing the SRT Workbook. You have learned new skills that will help you take control of your life and your illness. Remembering these important points will help you maintain stable social rhythms in the future:

- *Protect your body clock.* Body clocks affect many aspects of your physical and mental health, including sleep, hunger, energy, and mood. If you have bipolar disorder, you have a sensitive or fragile body clock. Keeping a regular schedule helps your body clock stay regular and contributes to mood stability.

- *Keep track of social rhythm anchors.* Your body clock is affected by cues in your environment, such as the time that you go to work or when you eat dinner. Be aware of these anchors and use them to keep your routines as regular as possible.

- *Keep track of social rhythm disruptors.* Social factors can disturb your body clock. For instance, going on vacation, traveling across time zones, and unexpected houseguests can throw your social rhythms into chaos. Keep alert for factors that may disrupt your routines and have a plan to get back on track with your schedule as quickly as possible.

- *Maintain good sleep habits.* Try to go to bed and get up at the same time every day—even on weekends!

- *Pay attention to light.* Light and dark have big impacts on body clocks. Be sure to get enough sunlight exposure during the daytime (aim for at least two hours a day) and good-quality darkness at night. Avoid blue spectrum light (emitted by virtually all screens and devices) in the evenings to optimize your sleep and circadian health. Keep your bedroom cool and dark.

- *Monitor your SRMs* regularly to detect changes in your mood and rhythms. If weekly feels like too much, consider completing it one week per month to keep an eye on your social rhythms. If your mood falters, get back on track by working on your SRM daily.

- *Work on communication.* Good communication improves relationships, which helps your routines and mood.

- *Keep others involved.* Educating close family and friends about your illness will have a positive impact on your health. Call them if you need them.

- *Know your early warning signs.* Keep your relapse prevention plan or a list of your possible warning signs handy to remind yourself of what to be on the lookout for. The better you know your warning signs, the more effective you'll be at detecting them when they show up in your life.

Additional resources. If you would like to learn more about circadian rhythms and brain health, here are some useful websites:

National Institute of Health: https://nigms.nih.gov/education/fact-sheets/Pages/circadian-rhythms.aspx

Enlighten Your Clock (comic book about circadian rhythms): https://enlightenyourclock.org/

Psych Education (reliable information about bipolar disorder): https://psycheducation.org/

Center for Environmental Therapeutics: https://cet.org

Self-guided IPSRT training program for therapists: https://ipsrt.org

Acknowledgments

Many individuals helped develop and refine Social Rhythm Therapy (SRT). Ellen Frank, the brilliant and innovative creator of Interpersonal and Social Rhythm Therapy (IPSRT), is the driving force behind SRT. I am enormously grateful to Dr. Frank, for more than twenty-five years of support and mentorship and her incomparable contributions to the field. Suffice it to say that SRT and this book would not exist without her.

SRT was honed over decades, with considerable input from therapists at the University of Pittsburgh. I wish to especially acknowledge Kelly Wells, Debra Frankel, and Kelly O'Toole, whose wisdom helped shape SRT. More recently, I have been honored to work with neuroimaging expert Hilary Blumberg and her team at Yale. Dr. Blumberg is studying neural circuitry changes associated with SRT, and I am grateful to her for taking SRT in this new direction. A big thank you to the Yale SRT therapists, Erin Carrubba and Bernadette Lecza, who helped refine the most recent version of the SRT manual, including providing thoughtful input about the impact of social media on daily routines.

I would like to thank those who offered critiques of earlier drafts of this workbook. I appreciate the constructive suggestions provided by my colleagues, Danielle Novick and Lauren Bylsma, as well as input from the New Harbinger editorial staff.

Finally, I would like to express gratitude to patients who entrusted me with their care and helped me understand why and how routines matter in bipolar disorder.

Social Rhythm Metric (SRM)

Directions:

- If desired, add two personalized activities in the blank boxes in the first column.

- Write the *ideal* target time you would *like* to do these daily activities (target time).

- Record the *time* you actually did the activity each day.

- Rate average mood and energy levels each day.

Date (week of): _____

Activity	Target Time	Sunday Time	Monday Time	Tuesday Time	Wednesday Time	Thursday Time	Friday Time	Saturday Time
Out of bed								
First contact with other person								
Start work/school/ volunteer/family care								
Dinner								
To bed								
Rate MOOD each day from −5 to +5 −5 = very depressed +5 = very elated								
Rate ENERGY LEVEL each day −5 = very slowed, fatigued +5 = very energetic, active								

References

Åkesson, S., M. Ilieva, J. Karagicheva, E. Rakhimberdiev, B. Tomotani, and B. Helm. 2017. "Timing Avian Long-Distance Migration: From Internal Clock Mechanisms to Global Flights." *Philosophical Transactions of the Royal Society of London. Series B, Biological Sciences* 372(1734): 20160252.

Altman, E. G., D. Hedeker, J. L. Peterson, and J. M. Davis. 1997. "The Altman Self-Rating Mania Scale." *Biological Psychiatry* 42(10): 948–955.

Andrabi, M., M. M. Andrabi, R. Kunjunni, M. K. Sriwastva, S. Bose, R. Sagar, et al. 2020. "Lithium Acts to Modulate Abnormalities at Behvioral, Cellular, and Molecular Levels in Sleep Deprivation-Induced Mania-Like Behavior." *Bipolar Disorders* 22(3): 266–80.

Ashman, S. B., T. H. Monk, D. J. Kupfer, C. H. Clark, F. S. Myers, E. Frank, et al. 1999. "Relationship Between Social Rhythms and Mood in Patients with Rapid Cycling Bipolar Disorder." *Psychiatry Research* 86(1): 1–8.

Bechtel, W. 2015. "Circadian Rhythms and Mood Disorders: Are the Phenomena and Mechanisms Causally Related?" *Frontiers in Psychiatry* 6: 118.

Belvederi Murri, M., D. Prestia, V. Mondelli, C. Pariante, S. Patti, B. Olivieri, et al. 2016. "The HPA Axis in Bipolar Disorder: Systematic Review and Meta-Analysis." *Psychoneuroendocrinology* 63: 327–42.

Benedetti, F., A. Serretti, C. Colombo, B. Barbini, C. Lorenzi, E. Campori, et al. 2003. "Influence of CLOCK Gene Polymorphism on Circadian Mood Fluctuation and Illness Recurrence in Bipolar Depression." *American Journal of Medical Genetics Part B, Neuropsychiatric Genetics: The Official Publication of the International Society of Psychiatric Genetics* 123B: 23–6.

Berk, M., S. Dodd, and G. S. Malhi. 2005. "'Bipolar Missed States': The Diagnosis and Clinical Salience of Bipolar Mixed States." *Australian & New Zealand Journal of Psychiatry* 39(4): 215–21.

Bishehsari, F., F. Levi, F. W. Turek, and A. Keshavarzian. 2016. "Circadian Rhythms in Gastrointestinal Health and Diseases." *Gastroenterology* 151(3): e1–5.

Bloch, G., E. D. Herzog, J. D. Levine, and W. J. Schwartz. 2013. "Socially Synchronized Circadian Oscillators." *Proceedings of the Royal Society B: Biological Sciences* 280(1765): 20130035.

Borbély, A. A. 1982. "A Two Process Model of Sleep Regulation." *Human Neurobiology* 1(3): 195–204.

Chong, P. L. H., D. Garic, M. D. Shen, I. Lundgaard, and A. J. Schwichtenberg. 2022. "Sleep, Cerebrospinal Fluid, and the Glymphatic System: A Systematic Review." *Sleep Medicine Reviews* 61: 101572.

Claustrat, B., J. Brun, and G. Chazot. 2005. "The Basic Physiology and Pathophysiology of Meltonin." *Sleep Medicine Reviews* 9(1): 11–24.

Colrain, I. M., C. L. Nicholas, and F. C. Baker. 2014. "Alcohol and the Sleeping Brain." *Handbook of Clinical Neurology* 125: 415–31.

Corruble, E., H. A. Swartz, T. Bottai, G. Vaiva, F. Bayle, P. M. Llorca, et al. 2016. "Telephone-Administered Psychotherapy in Combination with Antidepressant Medication for the Acute Treatment of Major Depressive Disorder." *Journal of Affective Disorders* 190: 6–11.

Coutrot, A., A. S. Lazar, M. Richards, E. Manley, J. M. Wiener, R. C. Dalton, et al. 2022. "Reported Sleep Duration Reveals Segmentation of the Adult Life-Course into Three Phases." *Nature Communications* 13: 7697.

Covassin, N., and P. Singh. 2016. "Sleep Duration and Cardiovascular Disease Risk: Epidemiologic and Experimental Evidence." *Sleep Medicine Clinics* 11(1): 81–9.

Crowe, M., M. Inder, H. A. Swartz, G. Murray, and R. Porter. 2020. "Social Rhythm Therapy—A Potentially Translatable Psychosocial Intervention for Bipolar Disorder." *Bipolar Disorders* 22(2): 121–7.

Dibner, C. 2020. "The Importance of Being Rhythmic: Living in Harmony with Your Body Clocks." *Acta Physiologica* 228(1): e13281.

Dresler, M., V. I. Spoormaker, P. Beitinger, M. Czisch, M. Kimura, A. Steiger, et al. 2014. "Neuroscience-Driven Discovery and Development of Sleep Therapeutics." *Pharmacology & Therapeutics* 141(3): 300–34.

Driver, H. S., and S. R. Taylor. 2000. "Exercise and Sleep." *Sleep Medicine Reviews* 4(4): 387–402.

Edgar, N., and C. A. McClung. 2013. "Major Depressive Disorder: A Loss of Circadian Synchrony?" *Bioessays* 35(11): 940–4.

Edinger, J. D., J. T. Arnedt, S. M. Bertisch, C. E. Carney, J. J. Harrington, K. L. Lichstein, et al. 2021. "Behavioral and Psychological Treatments for Chronic Insomnia Disorder in Adults: An American Academy of Sleep Medicine Clinical Practice Guideline." *Journal of Clinical Sleep Medicine* 17(2): 255–62.

Ehlers, C. L., D. J. Kupfer, E. Frank, and T. H. Monk. 1993. "Biological Rhythms and Depression: The Role of Zeitgebers and Zeitstorers." *Depression* 1(6): 285–93.

Eichhorn, G., M. P. Boom, H. P. van der Jeugd, A. Mulder, M. Wikelski, S. Maloney, et al. 2021. "Circadian and Seasonal Patterns of Body Temperature in Arctic Migratory and Temperate Non-Migratory Geese." *Frontiers in Ecology and Evolution* 9: 699917.

Ermer, A. E., and C. M. Proulx. 2022. "The Association Between Relationship Strain and Emotional Well-Being Among Older Adult Couples: The Moderating Role of Social Connectedness." *Aging & Mental Health* 26(6): 1198–1206.

Fares, S., D. F. Hermens, S. L. Naismith, D. White, I. B. Hickie, and R. Robillard. 2015. "Clinical Correlates of Chronotypes in Young Persons with Mental Disorders." *Chronobiology International* 32(9): 1183–91.

Flanagan, A., D. A. Bechtold, G. K. Pot, and J. D. Johnston. 2021. "Chrono-Nutrition: From Molecular and Neuronal Mechanisms to Human Epidemiology and Timed Feeding Patterns." *Journal of Neurochemistry* 157(1): 53–72.

Fowler, J. H., and N. A. Christakis. 2008. "Dynamic Spread of Happiness in a Large Social Network: Longitudinal Analysis over 20 Years in the Framingham Heart Study." *BMJ* 337: a2338.

Frank, E. 2005. *Treating Bipolar Disorder: A Clinician's Guide to Interpersonal and Social Rhythm Therapy*. New York: Guilford Press

Frank, E., D. J. Kupfer, M. Thase, A. Mallinger, H. A. Swartz, A. Fagiolini, et al. 2005. "Two-Year Outcomes for Interpersonal and Social Rhythm Therapy in Individuals with Bilpolar I Disorder." *Archives of General Psychiatry* 62(9): 996–1004.

Gariépy, G., H. Honkaniemi, and A. Quesnel-Vallée. 2016. "Social Support and Protection from Depression: Systematic Review of Current Findings in Western Countries." *The British Journal of Psychiatry: The Journal of Mental Science* 209(4): 284–93.

Gonzalez, R. 2014. "The Relationship Between Bipolar Disorder and Biological Rhythms." *Journal of Clinical Psychiatry* 75(4): e323–31.

Gottlieb, J. F., F. Benedetti, P. A. Geoffroy, T. E. G. Henriksen, R. W. Lam, G. Murray, et al. 2019. "The Chronotherapeutic Treatment of Bipolar Disorders: A Systematic Review and Practice Recommendations from the ISBD Task Force on Chronotherapy and Chronobiology." *Bipolar Disorders* 21(8): 741–73.

Harvey, A. G. 2008. "Sleep and Circadian Rhythms in Bipolar Disorder: Seeking Synchrony, Harmony, and Regulation." *The American Journal of Psychiatry* 165(7): 820–9.

Hester, L., D. Dang, C. J. Barker, M. Heath, S. Mesiya, T. Tienabeso, et al. 2021. "Evening Wear of Blue-Blocking Glasses for Sleep and Mood Disorders: A Systematic Review." *Chronobiology International* 38(10): 1375–83.

Hirschfeld, R. M., J. R. Calabrese, M. M. Weissman, M. Reed, M. A. Davies, M. A. Frye, et al. 2003. "Screening for Bipolar Disorder in the Community." *Journal of Clinical Psychiatry* 64(1): 53–9.

Hlastala, S. A. 2003. "Stress, Social Rhythms, and Behavioral Activation: Psychosocial Factors and the Bipolar Illness Course." *Current Psychiatry Reports* 5: 477–83.

Holt-Lunstad, J., T. F. Robles, and D. A. Sbarra. 2017. "Advancing Social Connection as a Public Health Priority in the United States." *American Psychologist* 72(6): 517–30.

Horne, J. A., and O. Ostberg. 1976. "A Self-Assessment Questionnaire to Determine Morningness-Eveningness in Human Circadian Rhythms." *International Journal of Chronobiology* 4(2): 97–110.

Johnston, J. D., J. M. Ordovás, F. A. Scheer, and F. W. Turek. 2016. "Circadian Rhythms, Metabolism, and Chrononutrition in Rodents and Humans." *Advances in Nutrition* 7(2): 399–406.

Jones, S. H., D. J. Hare, and K. Evershed. 2005. "Actigraphic Assessment of Circadian Activity and Sleep Patterns in Bipolar Disorder." *Bipolar Disorders* 7(2): 176–86.

Judd, L. L., P. J. Schettler, H. S. Akiskal, J. Maser, W. Coryell, D. Solomon, et al. 2003. "Long-Term Symptomatic Status of Bipolar I vs. Vipolar II Disorders." *Journal of Neuropsychopharmacology* 6(2): 127–37.

Kahawage, P., M. Crowe, J. Gottlieb, H. A. Swartz, L. N. Yatham, B. Bullock, et al. 2022. "Adrift in Time: The Subjective Experience of Circadian Challenge During COVID-19 Amongst People with Mood Disorders." *Chronobiology International* 39(1): 57–67.

Kalmbach, D. A., L. D. Schneider, J. Cheung, S. J Bertrand, T. Kariharan, A. I. Pack, et al. 2017. "Genetic Basis of Chronotype in Humans: Insights from Three Landmark GWAS." *Sleep* 40(2): zsw048.

Kolla, B. P., L. Hayes, C. Cox, L. Eatwell, M. Deyo-Svendsen, and M. P. Mansukhani. 2022. "The Effects of Cannabinoids on Sleep." *Journal of Primary Care & Community Health* 13: 21501319221081277.

Kraut, R., M. Patterson, V. Lundmark, S. Kiesler, T. Mukopadhyay, and W. Scherlis. 1998. "Internet Paradox: A Social Technology That Reduces Social Involvement and Psychological Well-Being?" *American Psychologist* 53(9): 1017–31.

Kroenke, K., R. L. Spitzer, and J. B. Williams. 2001. "The PHQ-9: Validity of a Brief Depression Severity Measure." *Journal of General Internal Medicine* 16(9): 606–13.

Kuhlman, S. J., L. M. Craig, and J. F. Duffy. 2018. "Introduction to Chronobiology." *Cold Spring Harbor Perspectives in Biology* 10(9): a033613.

Leigh-Hunt, N., D. Bagguley, K. Bash, V. Turner, S. Turnbull, N. Valtorta, et al. 2017. "An Overview of Systematic Review on the Public Health Consequences of Social Isolation and Loneliness." *Public Health* 152: 157–71.

Leverich, G. S., R. M. Post, P. E. Keck, Jr., L. L. Altshuler, M. A. Frye, R. W. Kupka, et al. 2007. "The Poor Prognosis of Childhood-Onset Bipolar Disorder." *The Journal of Pediatrics* 150(5): 485–90.

Liu, Y., A. G. Wheaton, D. P. Chapman, T. J. Cunningham, H. Lu, and J. B. Croft. 2016. "Prevalence of Healthy Sleep Duration Among Adults—United States, 2014." *MMWR Morbidity and Mortality Weekly Report* 65(6): 137–41.

Logan, R. W., and C. A. McClung. 2016. "Animal Models of Bipolar Mania: The Past, Present and Future." *Neuroscience* 321: 163–88.

———. 2019. "Rhythms of Life: Circadian Disruption and Brain Disorders Across the Lifespan," *Nature Reviews Neuroscience* 20: 49–65.

Lyall, L. M., C. A. Wyse, N. Graham, A. Ferguson, D. M. Lyall, B. Cullen, et al. 2018. "Association of Disrupted Circadian Rhythmicity with Mood Disorders, Subjective Wellbing, and Cognitive Function: A Cross-Sectional Study of 91 105 Participants from the UK Biobank." *Lancet Psychiatry* 5(6): 507–14.

Malkoff-Schwartz, S., E. Frank, B. Anderson, J. T. Sherrill, L. Siegel, D. Patterson, et al. 1998. "Stressful Life Events and Social Rhythm Disruption in the Onset of Manic and Depressive Bipolar Episodes." *Archives of General Psychiatry.* 55(8): 702–7.

Mansour, H. A., J. Wood, K. V. Chowdari, M. Dayal, M. E. Thase, D. J. Kupfer, et al. 2005. "Circadian Phase Variation in Bipolar I Disorder." *Chronobiology International* 22(3): 571–84.

Massar, S. A. A., J. Lim, and S. A. Huettel. 2019. "Sleep Deprivation, Effort Allocation and Performance." *Progress in Brain Research* 246: 1–26.

Maury, E., K. M. Ramsey, and J. Bass. 2010. "Circadian Rhythms and Metabolic Syndrome: From Experimental Genetics to Human Disease." *Circulation Research* 106(3): 447–62.

McCarthy, M. J., J. F. Gottlieb, R. Gonzalez, C. A. McClung, L. B. Alloy, S. Cain, et al. 2022. "Neurobiological and Behavioral Mechanisms of Circadian Rhythm Disruption in Bipolar Disorder: A Critical Multi-Disciplinary Literature Review and Agenda for Future Research from the ISBD Task Force on Chronobiology." *Bipolar Disorders* 24(3): 232–63.

McClung, C. A. 2007. "Circadian Genes, Rhythms and the Biology of Mood Disorders." *Pharmacology & Therapeutics* 114(2): 222–32.

———. 2013a. "How Might Circadian Rhythms Control Mood? Let Me Count the Ways." *Biological Psychiatry* 74(4): 242–9.

———. 2013b. "Mind Your Rhythms: An Important Role for Circadian Genes in Neuroprotection." *Journal of Clinical Investigation* 123(12): 4994–6.

Meng, J., X. Xiao, W. Wang, Y. Jiang, Y. Jin, and H. Wang. 2023. "Sleep Quality, Social Rhythms, and Depression Among People Living with HIV: A Path Analysis Based on Social Zeitgerber Theory." *Frontiers in Psychiatry* 14: 1102946.

Meyer, T. D., and S. Maier. 2006. "Is There Evidence for Social Rhythm Instability in People at Risk for Affective Disorders?" *Psychiatry Research* 141(1): 103–14.

Milhiet, V., B. Etain, C. Boudebesse, and F. Bellivier. 2011. "Circadian Biomarkers, Circadian Genes and Bipolar Disorders." *Journal of Physiology, Paris* 105(4–6): 183–9.

Mohr, D. C., P. Cuijpers, and K. Lehman. 2011. "Supportive Accountability: A Model for Providing Human Support to Enhance Adherence to eHealth Interventions." *Journal of Medical Internet Research* 13(1): e30.

Monk, T. H., E. Frank, J. M. Potts, and D. J. Kupfer. 2002. "A Simple Way to Measure Daily Lifestyle Regularity." *Journal of Sleep Research* 11(3): 183–90.

Monk, T. H., J. F. Flaherty, E. Frank, K. Hoskinson, and D. J. Kupfer. 1990. "The Social Rhythm Metric: An Instrument to Quantify the Daily Rhythms of Life." *Journal of Nervous and Mental Disease* 178(2): 120–6.

Monk, T. H., S. R. Petrie, A. J. Hayes, and D. J. Kupfer. 1994. "Regularity of Daily Life in Relation to Personality, Age, Gender, Sleep Quality and Circadian Rhythms." *Journal of Sleep Research* 3(4): 196–205.

Murray, G., and A. Harvey. 2010. "Circadian Rhythms and Sleep in Bipolar Disorder." *Bipolar Disorders* 12(5): 459–72.

Murray, G., J. Gottlieb, and H. A. Swartz. 2021. "Maintaining Daily Routines to Stabilize Mood: Theory, Data, and Potential Intervention for Circadian Consequences of COVID-19." *Canadian Journal of Psychiatry* 66(1): 9–13.

Nedeltcheva, A. V., and F. A. Scheer. 2014. "Metabolic Effects of Sleep Disruption, Links to Obesity and Diabetes." *Current Opinion in Endocrinology, Diabetes, Obesity* 21(4): 293–8.

Okamoto-Mizuno, K., and K. Mizuno. 2012. "Effects of Thermal Environment on Sleep and Circadian Rhythm." *Journal of Physiological Anthropology* 31(1): 14.

Paruthi, S., L. J. Brooks, C. D'Ambrosio, W. A. Hall, S. Kotagal, R. M. Lloyd, et al. 2016. "Consensus Statement of the American Academy of Sleep Medicine on the Recommended Amount of Sleep for Healthy Children: Methodology and Discussion." *Journal of Clinical Sleep Medicine* 12(11): 1549–61.

Portaluppi, F., R. Tiseo, M. H. Smolensky, R. C. Hermida, D. E. Ayala, and F. Fabbian. 2012. "Circadian Rhythms and Cardiovascular Health." *Sleep Medicine Reviews* 16(2): 151–66.

Sabet, S. M., N. D. Dautovich, and J. M. Dzierzewski. 2021. "The Rhythm Is Gonna Get You: Social Rhythms, Sleep, Depressive, and Anxiety Symptoms." *Journal of Affective Disorders* 286: 197–203.

Sankar, A., P. Panchal, D. A. Goldman, L. Colic, L. M. Villa, J. A. Kim, et al. 2021. "Telehealth Social Rhythm Therapy to Reduce Mood Symptoms and Suicide Risk Among Adolescents and Young Adults with Bipolar Disorder." *American Journal of Psychotherapy* 74(4): 172–7.

Saper, C. B., G. Cano, and T. E. Scammell. 2005. "Homeostatic, Circadian, and Emotional Regulation of Sleep." *The Journal of Comparative Neurology* 493(1): 92–8.

Savvidis, C., and M. Koutsilieris. 2012. "Circadian Rhythm Disruption in Cancer Biology." *Molecular Medicine* 18: 1249–60.

Schaffer, A., E. T. Isometsä, L. Tondo, D. H. Moreno, M. Sinyor, L. V. Kessing, et al. 2015. "Epidemiology, Neurobiology and Pharmacological Interventions Related to Suicide Deaths and Suicide Attempts in Bipolar Disorder: Part I of a Report of the International Society for Bipolar Disorders Task Force on Suicide in Bipolar Disorder." *The Australian & New Zealand Journal of Psychiatry* 49(9): 785–802.

Selmaoui, B., and Y. Touitou. 2003. "Reproducibility of the Circadian Rhythms of Serum Cortisol and Melatonin in Healthy Subjects: A Study of Three Different 24-H Cycles over Six Weeks." *Life Sciences* 73(26): 3339–49.

Shechter, A., E. W. Kim, M.-P. St-Onge, and A. J. Westwood. 2018. "Blocking Nocturnal Blue Light for Insomnia: A Randomized Controlled Trial." *Journal of Psychiatric Research* 96: 196–202.

Siwicki, K. K., P. E. Hardin, and J. L. Price. 2018. "Reflections on Contributing to 'Big Discoveries' About the Fly Clock: Our Fortunate Paths as Post-Docs with 2017 Nobel Laureates Jeff Hall, Michael Rosbash, and Mike Young." *Neurobiology of Sleep and Circadian Rhythms* 5: 58–67.

Skene, D. J., and J. Arendt. 2006. "Human Circadian Rhythms: Physiological and Therapeutic Relevance of Light and Melatonin." *Annals of Clinical Biochemistry* 43(Pt 5): 344–53.

Soreca, I., M. L. Wallace, E. Frank, B. P. Hasler, J. C. Levenson, and D. J. Kupfer. 2012. "Sleep Duration Is Associated with Dyslipidemia in Patients with Bipolar Disorder in Clinical Remission." *Journal of Affective Disorders* 141(0): 484–7.

Swartz, H. A., E. Frank, K. O'Toole, N. Newman, H. Kiderman, S. Carlson, et al. 2011. "Implementing Interpersonal and Social Rhythm Therapy for Mood Disorders Across a Continuum of Care." *Psychiatric Services* 62(11): 1377–80.

Swartz, H. A., P. Rucci, M. E. Thase, M. Wallace, E. Carretta, K. L. Celedonia, et al. 2018. "Psychotherapy Alone and Combined with Medication as Treatments for Bipolar II Depression: A Randomized Controlled Trial." *Journal of Clinial Psychiatry* 79: 7–15.

Sylvia, L. G., W. C. Chang, M. Kamali, M. Tohen, G. Kinrys, T. Deckersbach, et al. 2018. "Sleep Disturbance May Impact Treatment Outcome in Bipolar Disorder: A Preliminary Investigation in the Context of a Large Comparative Effectiveness Trial." *Journal of Affective Disorders* 225: 563–8.

Turek, F. W. 2016. "Circadian Clocks: Not Your Grandfather's Clock." *Science* 354(6315): 992–3.

Randler, C., C. Faßl, and N. Kalb. 2017. "From Lark to Owl: Developmental Changes in Morningness-Eveningness from New-Borns to Early Adulthood." *Scientific Reports* 7(45874): 1–8.

Roenneberg, T., A. Wirz-Justice, and M. Merrow. 2003. "Life Between Clocks: Daily Temporal Patterns of Human Chronotypes." *Journal of Biological Rhythms* 18(1): 80–90.

Roenneberg, T., and M. Merrow. 2007. "Entrainment of the Human Circadian Clock." *Cold Spring Harbor Symposia on Quantitative Biology* 72: 293–9.

Roenneberg, T., and R. J. Lucas. 2002. "Light, Endocrine Systems, and Cancer—A View from Circadian Biologists." *Neuro Endocrinology Letters* 23(Suppl 2): 82–3.

Vetter, C., D. Fischer, J. L. Matera, and T. Roenneberg. 2015. "Aligning Work and Circadian Time in Shift Workers Improves Sleep and Reduces Circadian Disruption." *Current Biology* 25(7): 907–11.

Vieta, E., M. Berk, T. G. Schultze, A. F. Carvalho, T. Suppes, J. R. Calabrese, et al. 2018. "Bipolar Disorders." *Nature Reviews Disease Primers* 4: 18008.

Wehrens, S. M. T., S. Christou, C. Isherwood, B. Middleton, M. A. Gibbs, S. N. Archer, et al. 2017. "Meal Timing Regulates the Human Circadian System." *Current Biology* 27(12): 1768–75.e3.

Weissman, M. M., J. C. Markowitz, and G. L. Klerman. 2018. *The Guide to Interpersonal Psychotherapy: Updated and Expanded Edition*. New York: Oxford University Press.

Wilhelm, I., J. Born, B. M. Kudielka, W. Schlotz, and S. Wüst. 2007. "Is the Cortisol Awakening Rise a Response to Awakening?" *Psychoneuroendocrinology* 32(4): 358–66.

World Health Organization. "International Statistical Classification of Diseases and Related Health Problems (ICD)." Accessed August 24, 2023. https://www.who.int/standards/classifications/classification-of-diseases.

Xie, L., H. Kang, Q. Xu, M. J. Chen, Y. Liao, M. Thiyagarajan, et al. 2013. "Sleep Drives Metabolite Clearance from the Adult Brain." *Science* 342(6156): 373–7.

Yatham, L. N., S. H. Kennedy, S. V. Parikh, A. Schaffer, D. J. Bond, B. N. Frey, et al. 2018. "Canadian Network for Mood and Anxiety Treatments (CANMAT) and International Society for Bipolar Disorders (ISBD) 2018 Guidelines for the Management of Patients with Bipolar Disorder." *Bipolar Disorders* 20(2): 97–170.

Zordan, M., R. Costa, G. Macino, C. Fukuhara, and G. Tosini. 2000. "Circadian Clocks: What Makes Them Tick?" *Chronobiology International* 17(4): 433–51.

Endnotes

1   M. J. McCarthy et al., 2022, "Neurobiological and Behavioral Mechanisms of Circadian Rhythm Disruption in Bipolar Disorder: A Critical Multi-Disciplinary Literature Review and Agenda for Future Research from the ISBD Task Force on Chronobiology," *Bipolar Disorders* 24(3): 232–63.

2   E. Frank, *Treating Bipolar Disorder: A Clinician's Guide to Interpersonal and Social Rhythm Therapy.* (New York: Guilford Press, 2005); E. Frank et al., 2005, "Two-Year Outcomes for Interpersonal and Social Rhythm Therapy in Individuals with Bilpolar I Disorder," *Archives of General Psychiatry* 62(9): 996–1004.

3   M. M. Weissman, J. C. Markowitz, and G. L. Klerman, *The Guide to Interpersonal Psychotherapy: Updated and Expanded Edition.* (New York: Oxford University Press, 2018).

4   L. N. Yatham et al., 2018, "Canadian Network for Mood and Anxiety Treatments (CANMAT) and International Society for Bipolar Disorders (ISBD) 2018 Guidelines for the Management of Patients with Bipolar Disorder," *Bipolar Disorders* 20(2): 97–170.

5   T. H. Monk et al., 2002, "A Simple Way to Measure Daily Lifestyle Regularity," *Journal of Sleep Research* 11(3): 183–90.

6   McCarthy et al., "Neurobiological and Behvioral Mechanisms," 232–63; F. Benedetti et al., 2003, "Influence of CLOCK Gene Polymorphism on Circadian Mood Fluctuation and Illness Recurrence in Bipolar Depression," *American Journal of Medical Genetics Part B, Neuropsychiatric Genetics: The Official Publication of the International Society of Psychiatric Genetics* 123B: 23–6.

7   C. A. McClung, 2007, "Circadian Genes, Rhythms and the Biology of Mood Disorders," *Pharmacology & Therapeutics* 114(2): 222–32.

8   Frank, *Treating Bipolar Disorder.*

9   Frank et al., "Two-Year Outcomes," 996–1004; J. F. Gottlieb et al., 2019, "The Chronotherapeutic Treatment of Bipolar Disorders: A Systematic Review and Practice Recommendations from the ISBD Task Force on Chronotherapy and Chronobiology," *Bipolar Disorders* 21(8): 741–73.

10 S. H. Jones et al., 2005, "Actigraphic Assessment of Circadian Activity and Sleep Patterns in Bipolar Disorder," *Bipolar Disorders* 7(2): 176–86.

11 McCarthy et al., "Neurobiological and Behvioral Mechanisms," 232–63.

12 C. A. McClung, 2013a, "How Might Circadian Rhythms Control Mood? Let Me Count the Ways," *Biological Psychiatry* 74(4): 242–9.

13 G. Murray, J. Gottlieb, and H. A. Swartz, 2021, "Maintaining Daily Routines to Stabilize Mood: Theory, Data, and Potential Intervention for Circadian Consequences of COVID–19." *Canadian Journal of Psychiatry* 66(1): 9–13.

14 V. Milhiet et al., 2011, "Circadian Biomarkers, Circadian Genes and Bipolar Disorders," *Journal of Physiology, Paris* 105(4–6): 183–9.

15 McCarthy et al., "Neurobiological and Behvioral Mechanisms," 232–63.

16 W. Bechtel, 2015, "Circadian Rhythms and Mood Disorders: Are the Phenomena and Mechanisms Causally Related?" *Frontiers in Psychiatry* 6: 118.

17 P. Kahawage et al., 2022, "Adrift in Time: The Subjective Experience of Circadian Challenge During COVID–19 Amongst People with Mood Disorders," *Chronobiology International* 39(1): 57–67; J. Meng et al., 2023, "Sleep Quality, Social Rhythms, and Depression Among People Living with HIV: A Path Analysis Based on Social Zeitgerber Theory," *Frontiers in Psychiatry* 14: 1102946.

18 F. W. Turek, 2016, "Circadian Clocks: Not Your Grandfather's Clock," *Science* 354(6315): 992–3.

19 S. J. Kuhlman, L. M. Craig, and J. F. Duffy, 2018, "Introduction to Chronobiology," *Cold Spring Harbor Perspectives in Biology* 10(9): a033613.

20   M. Zordan et al., 2000, "Circadian Clocks: What Makes Them Tick?," *Chronobiology International* 17(4): 433–51.

21   T. Roenneberg and M. Merrow, 2007, "Entertainment of the Human Circadian Clock," *Cold Spring Harbor Symposia on Quantitative Biology* 72: 293–9.

22   R. W. Logan and C. A. McClung, 2019, "Rhythms of Life: Circadian Disruption and Brain Disorders Across the Lifespan," *Nature Reviews Neuroscience* 20: 49–65.

23   R. Gonzalez, 2014, "The Relationship Between Bipolar Disorder and Biological Rhythms," *Journal of Clinical Psychiatry* 75(4): e323–31.

24   S. Fares et al., 2015, "Clinical Correlates of Chronotypes in Young Persons with Mental Disorders," *Chronobiology International* 32(9): 1183–91.

25   Turek, "Circadian Clocks," 992–3.

26   Logan and McClung, "Rhythms of Life," 49–65.

27   C. Dibner, 2020, "The Importance of Being Rhythmic: Living in Harmony with Your Body Clocks," *Acta Physiologica* 228(1): e13281.

28   S. M. T. Wehrens, 2017, "Meal Timing Regulates the Human Circadian System," *Current Biology* 27(12): 1768–75.

29   A. Flanagan et al., 2021, "Chrono-Nutrition: From Molecular and Neuronal Mechanisms to Human Epidemiology and Timed Feeding Patterns," *Journal of Neurochemistry* 157(1): 53–72.

30   K. K. Siwicki, P. E. Hardin, and J. L. Price, 2018, "Reflections on Contributing to 'Big Discoveries' About the Fly Clock: Our Fortunate Paths as Post–Docs with 2017 Nobel Laureates Jeff Hall, Michael Rosbash, and Mike Young," *Neurobiology of Sleep and Circadian Rhythms* 5: 58–67.

31   McClung, "Circadian Genes," 222–32.

32   M. Andrabi et al., 2020, "Lithium Acts to Modulate Abnormalities at Behvioral, Cellular, and Molecular Levels in Sleep Deprivation-Induced Mania–Like Behavior," *Bipolar Disorders* 22(3): 266–80.

33   R. W. Logan and C. A. McClung, 2016, "Animal Models of Bipolar Mania: The Past, Present and Future," *Neuroscience* 321: 163–88.

34   T. Roenneberg, A. Wirz-Justice, and M. Merrow, 2003, "Life Between Clocks: Daily Temporal Patterns of Human Chronotypes," *Journal of Biological Rhythms* 18(1): 80–90.

35   J. A. Home and O. Ostberg, 1976, "A Self-Assessment Questionnaire to Determine Morningness–Eveningness in Human Circadian Rhythms," *International Journal of Chronobiology* 4(2): 97–110.

36   D. A. Kalmbach et al., 2017, "Genetic Basis of Chronotype in Humans: Insights from Three Landmark GWAS," *Sleep* 40(2): zsw048.

37   C. Randler, C. Faßl, and N. Kalb, 2017, "From Lark to Owl: Developmental Changes in Morningness-Eveningness from New-Borns to Early Adulthood," *Scientific Reports* 7(45874): 1–8; T. H. Monk et al., 1994, "Regularity of Daily Life in Relation to Personality, Age, Gender, Sleep Quality and Circadian Rhythms," *Journal of Sleep Research* 3(4): 196–205.

38   H. A. Mansour et al., 2005, "Circadian Phase Variation in Bipolar I Disorder," *Chronobiology International* 22(3): 571–84.

39   Home and Ostberg, "A Self–Assessment Quiestionnaire," 97–110.

40   McCarthy et al., "Neurobiological and Behvioral Mechanisms," 232–63; McClung, "Circadian Genes," 222–32.

41   McClung, "Circadian Genes," 222–32.

42   McCarthy et al., "Neurobiological and Behvioral Mechanisms," 232–63.

43   Frank et al., "Two-Year Outcomes," 996–1004; H. A. Swartz et al., 2018, "Psychotherapy Alone and Combined with Medication as Treatments for Bipolar II Depression: A Randomized Controlled Trial," *Journal of Clinial Psychiatry* 79: 7–15.

44   M. Crowe et al., 2020, "Social Rhythm Therapy—A Potentially Translatable Psychosocial Intervention for Bipolar Disorder," *Bipolar Disorders* 22(2): 121–7.

45   T. H. Monk et al., 1990, "The Social Rhythm Metric: An Instrument to Quantify the Daily Rhythms of Life," *Journal of Nervous and Mental Disease* 178(2): 120–6.

46   S. A. Hlastala, 2003, "Stress, Social Rhythms, and Behavioral Activation: Psychosocial Factors and the Bipolar Illness Course," *Current Psychiatry Reports* 5: 477–83.

47   S. Malkoff–Schwartz et al., 1998, "Stressful Life Events and Social Rhythm Disruption in the Onset of Manic and Depressive Bipolar Episodes," *Archives of General Psychiatry*. 55(8): 702–7; S. B. Ashman et al., 1999, "Relationship Between Social Rhythms and Mood in Patients with Rapid Cycling Bipolar Disorder," *Psychiatry Research* 86(1): 1–8.

48   Murray, Gottlieb, and Swartz, "Maintaining Daily," 9–13; T. D. Meyer and S. Maier, 2006, "Is There Evidence for Social Rhythm Instability in People at Risk for Affective Disorders?" *Psychiatry Research* 141(1): 103–14.

49   Frank et al., "Two-Year Outcomes," 996–1004.

50   Monk et al., "The Social Rhythm Metric," 120–6.

51   Ibid.

52   Frank, *Treating Bipolar Disorder*; Monk et al., "A Simple Way," 183–90.

53   Frank, *Treating Bipolar Disorder*.

54   World Health Organization, "International Statistical Classification of Diseases and Related Health Problems (ICD)," accessed August 24, 2023, https://www.who.int/standards/classifications/classification–of–diseases.

55   E. Vieta et al., 2018, "Bipolar Disorders," *Nature Reviews Disease Primers* 4: 18008.

56   G. S. Leverich et al., 2007, "The Poor Prognosis of Childhood-Onset Bipolar Disorder," *The Journal of Pediatrics* 150(5): 485–90.

57   L. L. Judd et al., 2003, "Long-Term Symptomatic Status of Bipolar I vs. Vipolar II Disorders." *Journal of Neuropsychopharmacology* 6(2): 127–37.

58   Yatham et al., "Canadian Network," 97–170.

59   A. Sankar et al., 2021, "Telehealth Social Rhythm Therapy to Reduce Mood Symptoms and Suicide Risk Among Adolescents and Young Adults with Bipolar Disorder," *American Journal of Psychotherapy* 74(4): 172–7; H. A. Swartz et al., 2011, "Implementing Interpersonal and Social Rhythm Therapy for Mood Disorders Across a Continuum of Care," *Psychiatric Services* 62(11): 1377–80.

60   World Health Organization, "International Statistical Classification of Diseases and Related Health Problems (ICD)."

61   Ibid.

62   Ibid.

63   K. Kroenke, R. L. Spitzer, and J. B. Williams, 2001, "The PHQ–9: Validity of a Brief Depression Severity Measure," *Journal of General Internal Medicine* 16(9): 606–13.

64   A. Schaffer et al., 2015, "Epidemiology, Neurobiology and Pharmacological Interventions Related to Suicide Deaths and Suicide Attempts in Bipolar Disorder: Part I of a Report of the International Society for Biploar Disorders Task Force on Suicide in Bipolar Disorder," *The Australian & New Zealand Journal of Psychiatry* 49(9): 785–802.

65   World Health Organization, "International Statistical Classification of Diseases and Related Health Problems (ICD)."

66   Ibid.

67   E. G. Altman et al., 1997, "The Altman Self-Rating Mania Scale," *Biological Psychiatry* 42(10): 948–955.

68   R. M. Hirschfield et al., 2003, "Screening for Bipolar Disorder in the Community," *Journal of Clinical Psychiatry* 64(1): 53–9.

69   M. Berk, S. Dodd, and G. S. Malhi, 2005, "'Bipolar Missed States': The Diagnosis and Clinical Salience of Bipolar Mixed States," *Australian & New Zealand Journal of Psychiatry* 39(4): 215–21.

70   World Health Organization, "International Statistical Classification of Diseases and Related Health Problems (ICD)."

71   McCarthy et al., "Neurobiological and Behvioral Mechanisms," 232–63.

72   C. L. Ehlers et al., 1993, "Biological Rhythms and Depression: The Role of Zeitgebers and Zeitstorers." *Depression* 1(6): 285–93; N. Edgar and C. A. McClung, 2013, "Major Depressive Disorder: A Loss of Circadian Synchrony?" *Bioessays* 35(11): 940–4.

73   Crowe et al., "Social Rhythm Therapy," 121–7; E. Corruble et al., 2016, "Telephone-Administered Psychotherapy in Combination with Antidepressant Medication for the Acute Treatment of Major Depressive Disorder," *Journal of Affective Disorders* 190: 6–11.

74   Berk, Dodd, and Malhi, "Bipolar Missed States," 215–21.

75   Monk et al., "The Social Rhythm Metric," 120–6.

76   Monk et al., "A Simple Way," 183–90.

77   Frank et al., "Two-Year Outcomes," 996–1004.

78   S. M. Sabet, N. D. Dautovich, and J. M. Dzierzewski, 2021, "The Rhythm Is Gonna Get You: Social Rhythms, Sleep, Depressive, and Anxiety Symptoms," *Journal of Affective Disorders* 286: 197–203.

79   E. Maury, K. M. Ramsey, and J. Bass, 2010, "Circadian Rhythms and Metabolic Syndrome: From Experimental Genetics to Human Disease," *Circulation Research* 106(3): 447–62; C. A. McClung, 2013b, "Mind Your Rhythms: An Important Role for Circadian Genes in Neuroprotection," *Journal of Clinical Investigation* 123(12): 4994–6.

80   T. Roenneberg and R. J. Lucas, 2002, "Light, Endocrine Systems, and Cancer—A View from Circadian Biologists," *Neuro Endocrinology Letters* 23(Suppl 2): 82–3; C. Savvidas and M. Koutsileris, 2012, "Circadian Rhythm Disruption in Cancer Biology," *Molecular Medicine* 18: 1249–60.

81   F. Bishehsari et al., 2016, "Circadian Rhythms in Gastrointestinal Health and Diseases," *Gastroenterology* 151(3): e1–5.

82   J. D. Johnston et al., 2016, "Circadian Rhythms, Metabolism, and Chrononutrition in Rodents and Humans," *Advances in Nutrition* 7(2): 399–406.

83   Meng et al., "Sleep Quality," 1102946.

84   F. Portaluppi et al., 2012, "Circadian Rhythms and Cardiovascular Health," *Sleep Medicine Reviews* 16(2): 151–66.

85   D. C. Mohr, P. Cuijpers, and K. Lehman, 2011, "Supportive Accountability: A Model for Providing Human Support to Enhance Adherence to eHealth Interventions," *Journal of Medical Internet Research* 13(1): e30.

86   C. Vetter et al., 2015, "Aligning Work and Circadian Time in Shift Workers Improves Sleep and Reduces Circadian Disruption," *Current Biology* 25(7): 907–11.

87   A. G. Harvey, 2008, "Sleep and Circadian Rhythms in Bipolar Disorder: Seeking Synchrony, Harmony, and Regulation," *The American Journal of Psychiatry* 165(7): 820–9.

88   G. Murray and A. Harvey, 2010, "Circadian Rhythms and Sleep in Bipolar Disorder," *Bipolar Disorders* 12(5): 459–72; L. G. Sylvia et al., 2018, "Sleep Disturbance May Impact Treatment Outcome in Bipolar Disorder: A Preliminary Investigation in the Context of a Large Comparative Effectiveness Trial," *Journal of Affective Disorders* 225: 563–8.

89   M. Dresler et al., 2014, "Neuroscience-Driven Discovery and Development of Sleep Therapeutics," *Pharmacology & Therapeutics* 141(3): 300–34.

90   P. L. Chong et al., 2022, "Sleep, Cerebrospinal Fluid, and the Glymphatic System: A Systematic Review," *Sleep Medicine Reviews* 61: 101572.

91   I. Soreca et al., 2012, "Sleep Duration Is Associated with Dyslipidemia in Patients with Bipolar Disorder in Clinical Remission," *Journal of Affective Disorders* 141(0): 484–7.

92   Y. Liu et al., 2016, "Prevalence of Healthy Sleep Duration Among Adults—United States, 2014," *MMWR Morbidity and Mortality Weekly Report* 65(6): 137–41.

93   S. Paruthi et al., 2016, "Consensus Statement of the American Academy of Sleep Medicine on the Recommended Amount of Sleep for Healthy Children: Methodology and Discussion," *Journal of Clinical Sleep Medicine* 12(11): 1549–61.

94   A. Coutrot et al., 2022, "Reported Sleep Duration Reveals Segmentation of the Adult Life–Course into Three Phases," *Nature Communications* 13: 7697.

95   S. A. A. Massar, J. Lim, and S. A. Huettel, 2019, "Sleep Deprivation, Effort Allocation, and Performance," *Progress in Brain Research* 246: 1–26.

96   N. Covassin and P. Singh, 2016, "Sleep Duration and Cardiovascular Disease Risk: Epidemiologic and Experimental Evidence," *Sleep Medicine Clinics* 11(1): 81–9; A. V. Nedeltcheva and F. A. Scheer, 2014, "Metabolic Effects of Sleep Disruption, Links to Obesity and Diabetes," *Current Opinion in Endocrinology, Diabetes, Obesity* 21(4): 293–8.

97   B. Selmaoui and Y. Touitou, 2003, "Reproducibility of the Circadian Rhythms of Serum Cortisol and Melatonin in Healthy Subjects: A Study of Three Different 24–H Cycles over Six Weeks," *Life Sciences* 73(26): 3339–49.

98   Logan and McClung, "Rhythms of Life," 49–65.

99   D. J. Skene and J. Arendt, 2006, "Human Circadian Rhythms: Physiological and Therapeutic Relevance of Light and Melatonin," *Annals of Clinical Biochemistry* 43(5): 344–53.

100   I. Wilhelm et al., 2007, "Is the Cortisol Awakening Rise a Response to Awakening?," *Psychoneuroendocrinology* 32(4): 358–66.

101   B. Claustrat, J. Brun, and G. Chazot, 2005, "The Basic Physiology and Pathophysiology of Meltonin," *Sleep Medicine Reviews* 9(1): 11–24.

102   Milhiet et al., "Circadian Biomarkers," 183–9.

103   M. Belvederi Murri et al., 2016, "The HPA Axis in Bipolar Disorder: Systematic Review and Meta-Analysis," *Psychoneuroendocrinology* 63: 327–42.

104   L. Xie et al., 2013, "Sleep Drives Metabolite Clearance from the Adult Brain," *Science* 342(6156): 373–7.

105   C. B. Saper, G. Cano, and T. E. Scammel, 2005, "Homeostatic, Circadian, and Emotional Regulation of Sleep," *The Journal of Comparative Neurology* 493(1): 92–8.

106   A. A. Borbély, 1982, "A Two Process Model of Sleep Regulation," *Human Neurobiology* 1(3): 195–204.

107   I. M. Colrain, C. L. Nicholas, and F. C. Baker, 2014, "Alcohol and the Sleeping Brain," *Handbook of Clinical Neurology* 125: 415–31.

108   B. P. Kolla et al., 2022, "The Effects of Cannabinoids on Sleep," *Journal of Primary Care & Community Health* 13: 21501319221081277.

109   K. Okamoto–Mizuno and K. Mizuno, 2012, "Effects of Thermal Environment on Sleep and Circadian Rhythm," *Journal of Physiological Anthropology* 31(1): 14.

110   H. S. Driver and S. R. Taylor, 2000, "Exercise and Sleep," *Sleep Medicine Reviews* 4(4): 387–402.

111   A. Shechter et al., 2018, "Blocking Nocturnal Blue Light for Insomnia: A Randomized Controlled Trial," *Journal of Psychiatric Research* 96: 196–202.

112   L. Hester et al., 2021, "Evening Wear of Blue–Blocking Glasses for Sleep and Mood Disorders: A Systematic Review," *Chronobiology International* 38(10): 1375–83.

113   J. D. Edinger et al., 2021, "Behavioral and Psychological Treatments for Chronic Insomnia Disorder in Adults: An American Academy of Sleep Medicine Clinical Practice Guideline," *Journal of Clinical Sleep Medicine* 17(2): 255–62.

114   S. Åkesson et al., 2017, "Timing Avian Long-Distance Migration: From Internal Clock Mechanisms to Global Flights," *Philosophical Transactions of the Royal Society of London. Series B, Biological Sciences* 372(1734): 20160252.

115   G. Eichhorn et al., 2021, "Circadian and Seasonal Patterns of Body Temperature in Arctic Migratory and Temperate Non–Migratory Geese," *Frontiers in Ecology and Evolution* 9: 699917.

116   J. Holt–Lunstad, T. F. Robles, and D. A. Sbarra, 2017, "Advancing Social Connection as a Public Health Priority in the United States," *American Psychologist* 72(6): 517–30; R. Kraut et al., 1998, "Internet Paradox: A Social Technology That Reduces Social Involvement and Psychological Well-Being?," *American Psychologist* 53(9): 1017–31; G. Gariépy, H. Honkaniemi, and A. Quesnel-Vallée, 2016, "Social Support and Protection from Depression: Systematic Review of Current Findings in Western Countries," *The British Journal of Psychiatry: The Journal of Mental Science* 209(4): 284–93.

117   N. Leigh–Hunt et al., 2017, "An Overview of Systematic Review on the Public Health Consequences of Social Isolation and Loneliness," *Public Health* 152: 157–71.

118   J. H. Fowler and N. A. Christakis, 2008, "Dynamic Spread of Happiness in a Large Social Network: Longitudinal Analysis over 20 Years in the Framingham Heart Study," *BMJ* 337: a2338.

119   A. E. Ermer and C. M. Proulx, 2022, "The Association Between Relationship Strain and Emotional Well-Being Among Older Adult Couples: The Moderating Role of Social Connectedness," *Aging & Mental Health* 26(6): 1198–1206.

120   L. M. Lyall et al., 2018, "Association of Disrupted Circadian Rhythmicity with Mood Disorders, Subjective Wellbing, and Cognitive Function: A Cross–Sectional Study of 91 105 Participants from the UK Biobank," *Lancet Psychiatry* 5(6): 507–14.

121   G. Bloch et al., 2013, "Socially Synchronized Circadian Oscillators," *Proceedings of the Royal Society B: Biological Sciences* 280(1765): 20130035.

122   Covassin and Singh, "Sleep Duration and Cardiovascular Disease Risk," 81–9; Nedeltcheva and Scheer, "Metabolic Effects of Sleep Disruption," 293–8.

Holly A. Swartz, MD, is professor of psychiatry at the University of Pittsburgh School of Medicine, director of the Center for Advanced Psychotherapy, and an internationally recognized expert in psychosocial interventions for bipolar disorder. She is actively engaged in teaching, research, mentoring, and patient care. Swartz has held elected leadership positions for national and international professional organizations, including serving as president of the International Society of Interpersonal Psychotherapy, president of the International Society for Bipolar Disorders, and treasurer of the American Society of Clinical Psychopharmacology. She is author of more than one hundred publications, coeditor of *Bipolar II Disorder*, and editor in chief of the *American Journal of Psychotherapy*.

Foreword writer **Ellen Frank, PhD,** distinguished professor emeritus of psychiatry and psychology at the University of Pittsburgh School of Medicine, and cofounder and chief scientific officer at Health Rhythms, Inc.

Real change *is* possible

For more than forty-five years, New Harbinger has published proven-effective self-help books and pioneering workbooks to help readers of all ages and backgrounds improve mental health and well-being, and achieve lasting personal growth. In addition, our spirituality books offer profound guidance for deepening awareness and cultivating healing, self-discovery, and fulfillment.

Founded by psychologist Matthew McKay and Patrick Fanning, New Harbinger is proud to be an independent, employee-owned company. Our books reflect our core values of integrity, innovation, commitment, sustainability, compassion, and trust. Written by leaders in the field and recommended by therapists worldwide, New Harbinger books are practical, accessible, and provide real tools for real change.

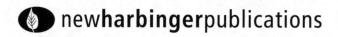 **newharbinger**publications

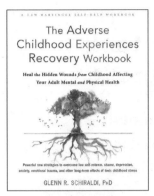
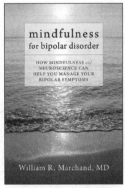
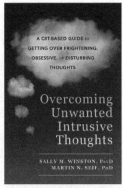
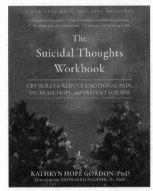
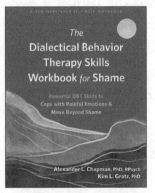
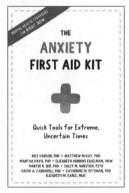

Did you know there are **free tools** you can download for this book?

Free tools are things like **worksheets**, **guided meditation exercises**, and **more** that will help you get the most out of your book.

You can download free tools for this book—whether you bought or borrowed it, in any format, from any source—from the New Harbinger website. All you need is a NewHarbinger.com account. Just use the URL provided in this book to view the free tools that are available for it. Then, click on the "download" button for the free tool you want, and follow the prompts that appear to log in to your NewHarbinger.com account and download the material.

You can also save the free tools for this book to your **Free Tools Library** so you can access them again anytime, just by logging in to your account! Just look for this button on the book's free tools page. ➜ **+ Save this to my free tools library**

If you need help accessing or downloading free tools, visit **newharbinger.com/faq** or contact us at **customerservice@newharbinger.com**.